Publisher CompletelyKeto Corp.

This publication is designed to provide authoritative information in regard to the subject matter covered. Many of the product designations are clarified by trademarks. While every precaution has been taken in the preparation of this book, the author assumes no responsibility for errors or omissions, or damages resulting from the use of information contained herein. For additional information, please contact our support team:

https://CompletelyKeto.com/support

202204043PFTFMP

Table of Contents

Sides 147

Fermented Veggies 163

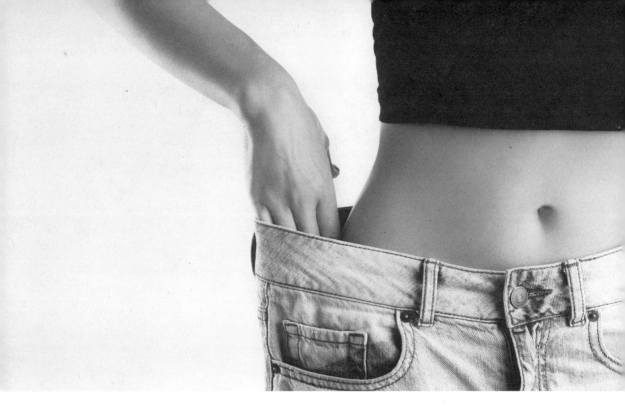

Disclaimer

Welcome and we're excited to have you with us on this journey. All of the information provided in the book and on the Websites located at completelyketo.com, completelyketo.shop, or speedketo.com or speedketo.shop is intended solely for general information and should NOT be relied upon for any particular diagnosis, treatment, or care. This book is not a substitute for medical advice. The book and websites are only for general informational purposes.

The information contained in this book is not a substitute for medical advice or treatment, and again the author strongly encourages patients and their families to consult with qualified medical professionals for treatment and related advice on individual cases.

Decisions relating to the prevention, detection, and treatment of all health issues should be made only after discussing the risks and benefits with your health care provider, considering your personal medical history, your current situation and your future health risks and concerns. If you are pregnant, nursing, diabetic, on medication, have a medical condition or are beginning a health or weight control program, consult your physician before using products or services discussed in this book and before making any other dietary changes. This diet is not recommended or supported for those under the age of eighteen. By using this book, you represent that you are at least eighteen (18) years old and a United States resident.

The authors cannot guarantee that the information in this book is safe and proper for every reader. For this reason, this book is offered without warranties or guarantees of any kind, expressed or implied, and the authors disclaim any liability, loss or damage caused by the contents, either directly or consequentially. The U.S. Food and Drug Administration or any other government regulatory body has not evaluated statements made in this book. Products, services, and methods discussed in this book are not intended to diagnose, treat, cure or prevent any disease.

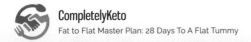

Introduction

The Belly Reset Diet

Babies are born with healthy tummies. When a baby eats, the system is so clean it rapidly comes out the other end.

But as the body gets older, the gut is affected. And the tummy grows and grows.

It doesn't have to be that way.

Legendary singer Elvis Presley died because his stomach and intestines were impacted after a lifetime of neglect. Eating white bread with peanut butter, bacon, butter and bananas took a toll.

If your tummy isn't what you want it to be, The Fat to Flat Masterplan is what you need.

I want you to start, right now by measuring your belly at its widest point.

Write that number down.

After the 28 days of following the program, I'll want you to measure again.

You'll be shocked at the results.

Our goal is to get that reset on your tummy so you can live your healthiest life ever.

- Harlan Kilstein Ed.D.

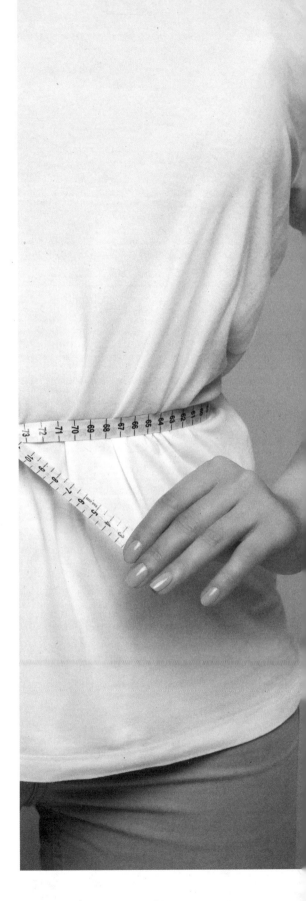

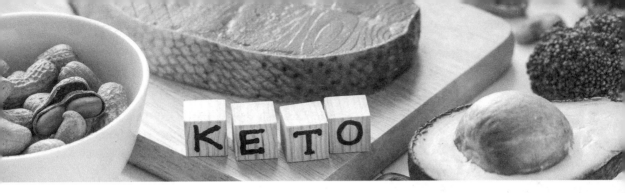

Chapter I: Fat to Flat Master Plan

Introduction

I've developed the new Fat to Flat Master Plan program to implement weight loss strategies that link the importance of a healthy digestive tract to efficient weight loss. While many of my clients have had easy success from following past programs there have been some that, despite compliance with the menu plan and a good effort, still experience slower weight loss than desired.

Over time I've found many in this group are also struggling with digestive issues such as:

- Acid reflux
- Gastroesophegeal Reflux Disease (GERD)
- Irritable Bowel Syndrome (IBS)
- Constipation or diarrhea
- Gas
- Bloating

New studies are finding potential links between the gut microbiome and successful weight loss for dieters. But before we get into this, first let me give you a quick synopsis of how a ketogenic diet can work for weight-loss.

How a ketogenic eating plan works

Carbohydrates are a macronutrient (macro) your body uses to create energy. Once ingested, all carbohydrates are broken down during the digestion process into smaller sugar units which are then absorbed through the intestinal wall into the bloodstream. When they reach the liver they are converted into glucose and carried to all parts of the body by insulin. Glucose can be used by every cell of the body for energy and this is where insulin becomes necessary.

In order for glucose to be transferred into a body cell, insulin has to connect to a special receptor on the wall of the cell. Here it acts like a key fitting into a lock, to open up the cell so the glucose molecule can enter and be used as energy. Glucose is then used for basic bodily functions like breathing and muscle power during physical activity.

If glucose isn't used right away the liver will convert the excess glucose into glycogen which can be stored in the liver and large skeletal muscles. But there's a limit to how much glycogen can be stored at one time and that's about 2,000 calories worth. If a large amount of carbohydrate has been consumed, the extra glucose produced will be stored as body fat!

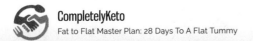

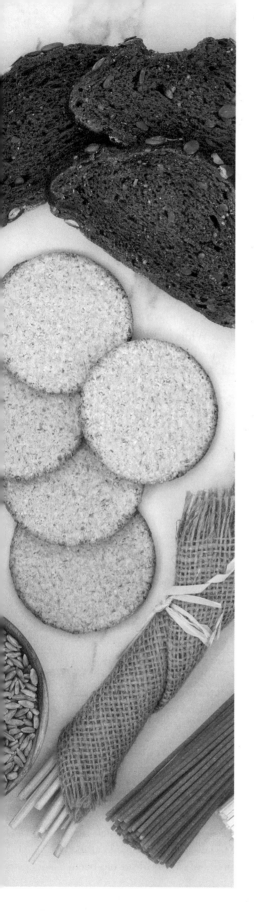

Carbohydrates come in two forms:

- Simple carbohydrates: contain less than three molecules and take less time to digest so they are absorbed quickly and lead to a quick burst of energy (a sugar "high").

- Complex carbohydrates: contain three or more molecules and take longer to digest. Vegetables, whole grains and foods we sometimes call starches, like potatoes all contain complex carbohydrates.

It's easy to over-consume carbs even if you abstain from sugar. What may seem like healthy choices, whole grains, breads (even when made using whole wheat and other whole grains), rice and fruits are all full of carbohydrates.

Once you eat them they are broken down during the digestion process and made into glucose ready for use or storage. If not burned off they are converted and stored as body fat for later use. Complex carbs are just longer chains of glucose molecules … once ingested and digested they become sugar in the blood.

A ketogenic eating plan, like this Fat to Flat Master Plan program, purposefully limits the amount of carbohydrates consumed while allowing for the consumption of moderate amounts of protein and a higher consumption of fats. This allows the liver to break down stored body fat into a source of energy the body can easily use called ketone bodies. When the amount of carbohydrates consumed daily is limited, the body is forced to use this alternative metabolic process, called ketosis, to create energy.

Now that you have a basic understanding of how a ketogenic eating program works to promote weight loss, let me take a deeper dive into the thinking and research behind this new Fat to Flat Master Plan program.

What is meant by "gut microbiome"?

Bacteria, viruses and fungi are collectively known as micro-organisms or microbes for short. Many live in and on your body. There are trillions (yes trillions!) of them at any given time that are alive and sharing, in a very intimate way, your personal space.

Bacterial microbes live in the large intestine and are mostly located in an area called the cecum. When food exits the stomach it first travels through the small intestine but is only partially digested as it reaches the first part of the large intestine. This is the area known as the cecum.

Anatomy of Intestine

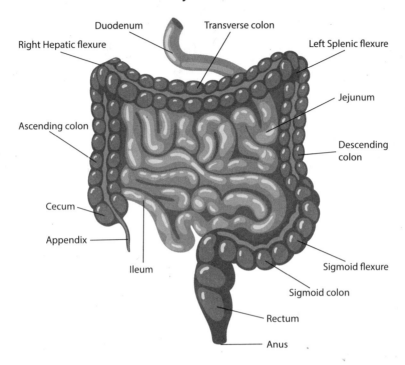

It is a long tube-like section, slightly wider and more pouch-like than the remaining part of the large intestine and is located in the lower right side of the abdomen, at the bottom of the upright colon. The bacteria that make their home here, apparently over 1,000 different species,[1] are what we are referring to when we talk about the gut microbiome.

"Good" bacteria and "bad" bacteria

As we know some bacteria cause disease and others are beneficial to your health. These "good" bacteria work in harmony with your body to:

- maintain heart health
- support a strongly functioning immune system
- maintain healthy skin
- support Brain health
- support and maintain a healthy mouth environment
- maintain and support a healthy body weight

These are only a few examples of how your microbiome works to keep you healthy. We really don't know all there is to know about these micro-organisms that coordinate with our own bodily systems but research is ongoing and recent findings are of great interest to those who struggle in their efforts to lose weight. The majority of these studies focus on various types of bacteria.

1 Ron Sender, Shai Fuchs, Ron Milo. *Revised Estimates for the Number of Human and Bacteria Cells in the Body* PLoS Biol. 2016 Aug; 14(8): e1002533. Published online 2016 Aug 19. doi: 10.1371/journal.pbio.1002533. Retrieved from https://www.cancer.gov/publications/dictionaries/cancer-terms/def/cecum on 2022/03/02.

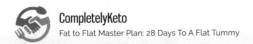

These bacteria break food down into components your body can use. But they also have other important work to accomplish. "Good" bacteria work to keep the "bad" bacteria (the ones that cause disease) in check by multiplying so efficiently they simply outnumber the troublesome bad bacteria.[2] If the gut microbiome is unbalanced, a larger number of the bad bacteria can leak through the intestinal lining into the body where the immune system kicks into action to curtail their affect on the body.

An immune system that's constantly being activated in this way can lead to wide-spread inflammation which, in turn, can make weight-loss grind to halt.[3] While imbalance in the gut microbiome is only one of the factors that contribute to inflammation in the body, it is important to note. Making an effort to correct the situation is important too. While research continues that delves more deeply into the role that the gut microbiome plays in general health and more specifically in maintaining a healthy body weight there are steps you can take today to promote weight loss. This new Fat to Flat Master Plan program is aimed at creating an environment in the intestines that encourages a healthy gut microbiome.

Weight gain and your gut...

The many different species of good bacteria living in the intestines all have a different genetic make-up and all have a different effect in the gut microbiome.

A study, published in the American Society for Microbiology (ASM) journal in September, 2021, looked at the genetic make-up of gut bacteria in a small group of dieters. Some of the dieters experienced successful weight-loss with a controlled weight loss program while others did not. Differences in the genetic make-up of the gut microbiome in the successful participants when compared to those of the unsuccessful were identified and might contain important information for those struggling to lose weight.[4] The genus, *Prevotella* was noted as being present in greater numbers for the dieters who experienced the most weight loss.

This study included only a small number of subjects so the results need to be replicated with a much larger group. Perhaps, based on studies such as this one cited here, probiotic supplements will be available in the future, specifically formulated for weight loss.

In the meantime I am recommending that my clients include a good quality probiotic in their daily supplementation regime. I also outline a daily menu plan that includes a variety of fermented foods which also contribute "good" bacteria to aid in establishing a healthy gut microbiome. Fermented foods are so important I've given them a *whole chapter* of their own!

In order to feed and maintain the "good" bacteria of the gut microbiome regular consumption of high fiber foods is also a must.

2 Hjorth, M.F., Blædel, T., Bendtsen, L.Q. et al. *Prevotella-to-Bacteroides* ratio predicts body weight and fat loss success on 24-week diets varying in macronutrient composition and dietary fiber: results from a post-hoc analysis. Int J Obes 43, 149–157 (2019). Retrieved from https://doi.org/10.1038/s41366-018-0093-2. on 2022/03/02

3 Author: Jennifer luz Medical Reviewer: Jessica Rodriguez. *Obesity and Inflammation: A Vicious Cycle.* Retrieved from https://www.endocrineweb.com/obesity-inflammation-cycle on 2022/03/03

4 Christian Diener, Shizhen Qin, Yong Zhou, Sushmita Patwardhan, Li Tang, Jennifer C. Lovejoy, Andrew T. Magis, Nathan D. Price, Leroy Hood, Sean M. Gibbons. *Baseline Gut Metagenomic Functional Gene Signature Associated with Variable Weight Loss Responses* following a Healthy Lifestyle Intervention in Humans. ASM Journals Systems Vol. 6, No. 5. Retrieved from https://journals.asm.org/doi/10.1128/mSystems.00964-21 on 2022/03/02

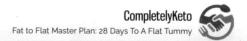

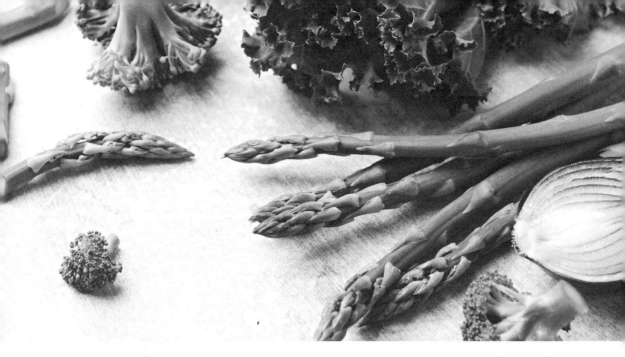

The importance of high fiber foods...

The digestive process begins in the mouth where saliva mixes with food as you chew before swallowing. Digestion continues in the stomach and then the small intestine but the fiber in your diet doesn't get broken down until it reaches the large intestine (the colon). Here, depending on the type of fiber, it's either fermented by bacteria or continues along the length of the colon and is eliminated as stool (feces). There are two types of fiber: soluble and insoluble. Both are important for different reasons.

Insoluble fiber does not get digested but works to provide bulk to stools making them easier to move along through the colon and helping to alleviate or prevent constipation. Its bulkiness may also work to create a feeling of fullness for a longer period of time, making it easier to eat less and resist snacking between meals.

Remember the "good" bacteria in the cecum, the pouch located at the beginning of the large colon? Bacteria here work to ferment soluble fiber. We need these bacteria as our bodies are incapable of digesting fiber without their help and we need the benefit of soluble fiber:

- Evidence shows that soluble fiber helps control blood sugar making it important for clients with Type 2 diabetes.[5]

- Soluble fiber has also been shown to alleviate symptoms of IBS.[6]

In this program a carefully selected variety of veggies, berries and some seeds bring fiber into your daily food consumption without making the net carb count so high it kicks you out of ketosis. Here's a list of 12 fruits, vegetables and seeds that you will see repeated on the four week menu plan along with their net carbs and fiber counts:

5 Jovanovski E, Khayyat R, Zurbau A, Komishon A, Mazhar N, Sievenpiper JL, Blanco Mejia S, Ho HVT, Li D, Jenkins AL, Duvnjak L, Vuksan V. *Should Viscous Fiber Supplements Be Considered in Diabetes Control? Results From a Systematic Review and Meta-analysis of Randomized Controlled Trials.* Diabetes Care. 2019 May;42(5):755-766. doi: 10.2337/dc18-1126. Epub 2019 Jan 7. Erratum in: Diabetes Care. 2019 Aug;42(8):1604. PMID: 30617143. Retrieved from https://pubmed.ncbi.nlm.nih.gov/30617143/ on 2022/03/04

6 Moayyedi P, Quigley EM, Lacy BE, Lembo AJ, Saito YA, Schiller LR, Soffer EE, Spiegel BM, Ford AC. *The effect of fiber supplementation on irritable bowel syndrome: a systematic review and meta-analysis.* Am J Gastroenterol. 2014 Sep;109(9):1367-74. doi: 10.1038/ajg.2014.195. Epub 2014 Jul 29. PMID: 25070054. Retrieved from https://pubmed.ncbi.nlm.nih.gov/25070054/ on 2022/03/04

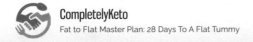

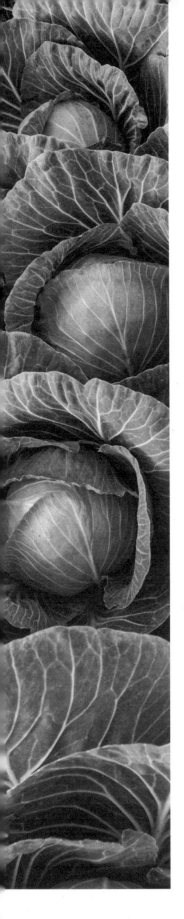

- Avocado: one medium sized avocado contains less than 4g of net carbs and almost 14g of fiber
- Collard: 1 C of chopped and cooked collard greens contain only 3 g of net carbs and 8g of fiber
- Chia seeds: 1 T provide only 1g of net carbs and a whopping 6g of fiber
- Raspberries: ½ C provides 3g of net carbs and 4g of fiber
- Blackberries: ½ C provides 3g of net carbs and 4g of fiber
- Artichoke: if you eat only the edible part at the base of one medium sized artichoke (the heart) you get 1 g net carbs and 3g of fiber
- Cabbage: 1 C shredded cabbage has 1g net carbs and 2G of fiber
- Flax seed: 1 T ground flax seed has 0 carbs and 2g of fiber
- Broccoli: 1 C florets have 4g net carbs and 2g of fiber
- Cauliflower: 1 C of florets have about 3g of net carbs and 2g of fiber
- Kale: 1 C yields 4g net carbs and 2g fiber
- Asparagus: a serving of 6 medium spears yield 2g net carbs and 2g fiber

White fat and brown fat

Inside our bodies we have both white adipose tissue (white fat) and brown adipose tissue (brown fat).

I've already covered how excess glucose is transported throughout the body and stored inside white fat cells in the form of lipids, with the aid of insulin. White adipose tissue is found in and around internal organs and also under the skin.

Bears stay warm during hibernation periods because they have a large amount of brown adipose tissue, commonly referred to as brown fat. Our bodies have brown fat too. Babies are born with significant deposits of brown fat to help them keep warm when they first emerge into the world. The ability to shiver isn't developed right away and the brown fat in their little bodies allows them to produce heat when they are cold.

While a white fat cell is full of energy stored as lipids, brown fat is packed with mitochondria. Mitochondria have a high iron content which gives this type of fat its brownish color. It is the large amount of mitochondria that turn these cells into tiny and efficient, heat producing furnaces.

This sizeable, brown fat deposit in newborns is situated on the baby's back in the area of the upper spine, between the shoulder blades and in the back of the neck. The brown fat here actually produces heat inside the body when activated. The ability to shiver eventually develops in an infant and the size of the brown fat deposit diminishes over time.

Adults still have a residual amount of brown fat in this same area, as it never completely disappears. Adults also have brown fat in small amounts located in various other locations throughout the body.[7]

Recruitable brown fat

In 2013 two separate teams of scientists, funded by NIH research, gave us additional information about brown fat function in mice. As a result of their work two distinct types of brown fat have been described. The type of brown fat present at birth is called constitutive brown fat but there is a second type that can actually be created called recruitable brown fat. It turns out white adipose tissue can be changed into brown fat. When certain proteins are present they can trigger white cells to become brown fat cells. This recruitable brown fat is found in small amounts throughout white fat deposits and muscle tissue.[8]

Since 2013 numerous other studies have been conducted that confirm the presence of recruitable brown adipose tissue in people. We know a brown fat cell is packed with mitochondria that turn it into a furnace, burning calories to create heat. But ... where do they get the calories to burn? Well, the obvious answer is from the lipids stored inside white fat cells, located close by.

Can we create an environment, by using specific interventions, where white fat cells will change into even more recruitable brown fat cells; all cannibalizing even more white fat cells for energy? For the last decade, in an effort to find effective interventions and treatments for the obesity epidemic plaguing the country, researchers have been conducting studies to answer this and other similar questions.[9,10,11]

Easy to implement interventions to boost brown fat activity...

- Men exposed to a cool environment overnight for a month had an increase in brown fat with corresponding changes in metabolism.[9] The take-away here is one that is easy to implement. *Sleep in a cool room (at or below 66 F).*

- When the temperatures around you are lower your body makes more recruitable brown fat so make sure to continue taking *daily walks during the winter months.*

- People who engage in cardio-vascular work-outs have a higher percentage of brown fat in their bodies. If you are able, develop a vigorous exercise program. I encourage daily walking, so *make it a brisk walk*, if you can.

- Eating and drinking thermogenic foods has been shown to promote weight loss by stimulating brown fat activity.[11] I provide five different teas, known to increase metabolism, on the daily menu plan. Make sure to *drink the teas* as suggested.

---

7 Author: Harrison Wein, Ph.D. *Overlooked "Brown Fat" Tied to Obesity.* Retrieved from, https://www.nih.gov/news-events/nih-research-matters/overlooked-brown-fat-tied-obesity on 2022/03/06

8 Author: Dr. Francis Collins. *Brown Fat, White Fat, Good Fat, Bad Fat.* Retrieved from https://directorsblog.nih.gov/2013/03/26/brown-fat-white-fat-good-fat-bad-fat/ on 2022/03/06

9 Author: Carol Torgan, Ph.D *Cool Temperature Alters Human Fat and Metabolism.* Retrieved from https://www.nih.gov/news-events/nih-research-matters/cool-temperature-alters-human-fat-metabolism on 2022/03/06

10 Author: Carol Torgan, Ph.D. *Insights into Energy-Burning Fat Cells* retrieved from https://www.nih.gov/news-events/nih-research-matters/insights-into-energy-burning-fat-cells on 2022/03/06

11 Masayuki Saito, Mami Matsushita, Takeshi Yoneshiro, Yuko Okamatsu-Ogura. *Brown Adipose Tissue, Diet-Induced Thermogenesis, and Thermogenic Food Ingredients: From Mice to Men.* Retrieved from https://www.ncbi.nlm.nih.gov/pmc/articles/PMC7186310/ on 2022/03/06

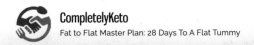

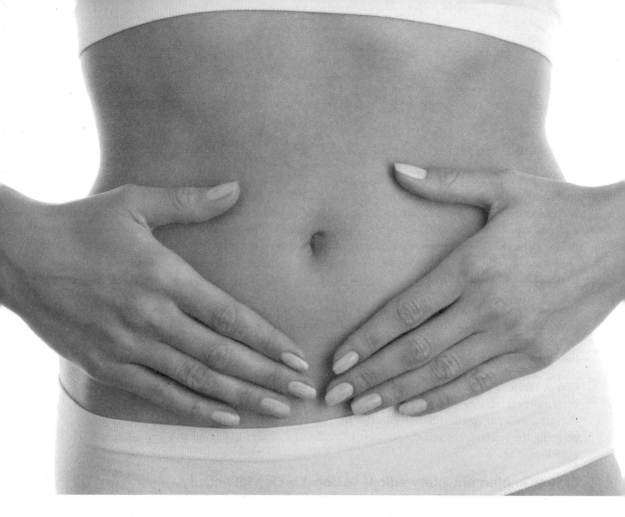

Why it's important to flatten your tummy...

While sedentary people who are overweight have an increased chance of developing pre-diabetes and eventually Type 2 diabetes it's interesting to note there are many over-weight people who do *not* become insulin resistant. Similarly there are also slim people who *do* develop insulin resistance and go on to eventually be diagnosed with Type 2 diabetes. So what's at play here?

It turns out where you carry your excess weight makes a difference. When the majority of excess pounds are packed in around the trunk of the body (visceral fat) as opposed to being more evenly distributed around the rest of the body and deposited just beneath the skin (subcutaneous fat), there is a corresponding higher risk of developing insulin resistance and eventual Type 2 diabetes.

Visceral fat

Visceral fat isn't always obvious. Just a slightly thicker waistline could be hiding fat packed in and around internal organs. This explains how some normal weight people can be afflicted with Type 2 diabetes.[2]

There are two types of visceral fat:

- Omental fat: found outside and around the internal organs of the abdomen (liver, kidneys, pancreas, stomach and intestines).

- Intra-organic fat: These deposits of fat are actually *inside* the organs

 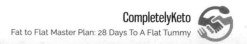

Stages of Liver Damage

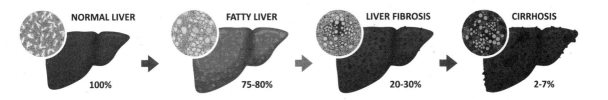

NORMAL LIVER 100% → FATTY LIVER 75-80% → LIVER FIBROSIS 20-30% → CIRRHOSIS 2-7%

Fatty liver, fatty muscles, fatty pancreas

Let's take a closer look at what's happening when excess weight starts to accumulate in the trunk of the body. The first place this intra-organic fat starts to show up is in the liver.

When the liver has created the maximum amount of glycogen that it can store it switches into transforming glucose (and to a lesser extent protein) into fat molecules which are then shipped out to fat cells, wherever they happen to be, for storage as body fat. For people who tend to pack the pounds on subcutaneously there doesn't seem to be too much of a metabolic issue, at least not until the abdomen starts to enlarge. But for the folks who carry most of their excess weight around the middle, fat storage becomes an issue much sooner

Since the liver is the site where glucose is processed it makes sense that the organ affected with internal fat deposits first would be the liver. This is how Dr. Fung, a Canadian nephrologist, describes the process:

1. Hyperinsulinemia causes fatty liver
2. Fatty liver causes insulin resistance
3. Insulin resistance leads to compensatory Hyperinsulinemia
4. Cycle repeats[12]

He goes on to say "fat inside the liver, rather than over-all obesity, is the crucial stepping stone towards insulin resistance and diabetes."[13]

It isn't just the liver that gets "fatty". A similar thing happens in the muscles too, according to Dr. Fung. He calls it Fatty Muscles. The human body can accumulate lines of fat looking much like those marbled steaks we love to eat! The end result isn't as pretty ... as fat accumulates these big skeletal muscle groups also become insulin resistant.[14]

And the process continues until eventually the pancreas becomes riddled with deposits of fatty tissue.

---

12 Fung, Jason MD, *The Diabetes Code: Prevent and Reverse Diabetes Naturally.* Location 1330, Greystone Books, Vancouver/Berkley,

13 Fung, Jason MD, *The Diabetes Code: Prevent and Reverse Diabetes Naturally.* Chapter 7: Diabetes a Disease of Dual Defects. Location 1330. Greystone Books, Vancouver/Berkley

14 Fung, Jason MD, *The Diabetes Code: Prevent and Reverse Diabetes Naturally.* Chapter 7: Diabetes a Disease of Dual Defects. Location 1408 – 1434. Greystone Books, Vancouver/Berkley

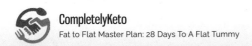

Pancreatic beta cell dysfunction

This instigates the second phase in the process that leads to Type 2 diabetes as described by Dr. Fung: "In the second phase, fatty pancreas creates beta cell dysfunction. The pancreas is not burnt out; it is merely clogged with fat."[15]

As the pancreas becomes increasingly riddled with fat deposits its groupings of beta cells are simply unable to produce adequate insulin. For many years this condition was considered to be irreversible however we now know this to be untrue.

A 2011 study, published first in Diabetologia, included 11 patients with Type 2 diabetes as well as a control group without this disease. They were all put on a very restricted, low calorie diet of only 600 calories/day. After just one week fasting plasma glucose normalized in the Type 2 diabetes group.

By the end of the 8 week study the scientists involved were able to conclude: "Normalization of both beta cell function and hepatic insulin sensitivity in Type 2 diabetes was achieved by dietary energy restriction alone. This was associated with decreased pancreatic and liver triacylglycerol stores. The abnormalities underlying Type 2 diabetes are reversible by reducing dietary energy intake."[16]

So, Type 2 diabetes can be reversed; the pancreas can recover and function normally again ... given the right treatment.

What are leptins and what do they do?

Leptin is commonly known as the hunger hormone. Much of the leptin that circulates in the bloodstream is produced by adipose tissue (fat cells) and seems to be the main way that these cells communicate directly with the brain. When a larger amount of leptin is released into the blood your fat cells are communicating how much energy is stored inside them in the form of lipids. Based on this information from the fat cells, the brain will know you aren't starving and will signal satiety. This means you will feel full.

Conversely, when leptin levels drop the brain signals hunger and you are prompted to eat more.[17] If the brain senses low leptin on a continual basis the body's metabolic rate will be also be lowered as the brain now goes into starvation mode and works to limit how the body will use its limited store of energy; the end result being weight loss slows down or stops.

Leptin, obesity and leptin resistance

If you have struggled with being overweight you are familiar with the shaming that our culture heaps upon those wanting desperately to lose those excess pounds. "Just push away from the table" thinking serves only to make the situation worse. Over the past two decades many scientific studies have focused on the role the hormone leptin plays in obesity. It's known as the "hunger" hormone because one of its functions in the body is to signal the brain when it's time to eat and stimulates the feeling we all know as hunger.

15 Fung, Jason MD, *The Diabetes Code: Prevent and Reverse Diabetes Naturally.* Chapter 7: Diabetes a Disease of Dual Defects. Location 1483. Greystone Books, Vancouver/Berkley

16 Lim, E.L., Hollingsworth, K.G., Aribisala, B.S. et al. *Reversal of type 2 diabetes: normalisation of beta cell function in association with decreased pancreas and liver triacylglycerol Diabetologia* (2011) 54: 2506. Retrieved from https://doi.org/10.1007/s00125-011-2204-7 Retrieved on: 09/05/2018

17 Chan JL, Heist K, DePaoli AM, Veldhuis JD, Mantzoros CS. *The role of falling leptin levels in the neuroendocrine and metabolic adaptation to short-term starvation in healthy men.* J Clin Invest. 2003 May;111(9):1409-21. doi: 10.1172/JCI17490. Retrieved from https://pubmed.ncbi.nlm.nih.gov/12727933/ on 2022/03/08

CompletelyKeto
Fat to Flat Master Plan: 28 Days To A Flat Tummy

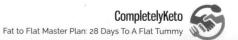

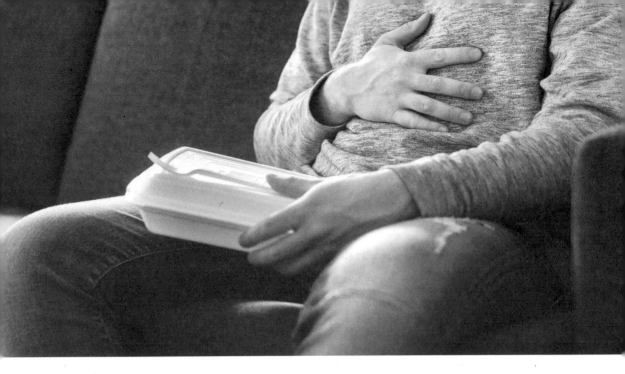

When leptin levels drop in the bloodstream we feel hunger and when they rise the brain tells us we are full by feelings of satiety. When leptin was first recognized as being a critical part of the hunger response system in 1994, it was thought that obese people may be predisposed to weight gain because they simply didn't make enough leptin. Perhaps low levels of leptin in the bloodstream meant the brain wasn't getting stimulated to send the "I'm full, stop eating" signal.

With more study it was shown that the majority of obese individuals actually had sufficient levels of leptin circulating for the "I'm full" signal to be triggered. It seemed that even though adequate leptin was available the signal wasn't getting into the brain. The end result being overeating, a lowered metabolic rate with weight gain and obesity being the outcome. So, the next question became what is causing this leptin resistance?[18]

The brain is protected by something called the blood brain barrier (BBB). This barrier surrounds the vascular system inside the brain and is made up of different types of cells. These cells work together to protect the brain by regulating what can pass through them and into the central nervous system from the bloodstream.[19]

Since leptin levels in the blood are usually high enough in the obese to be signaling the brain that starvation isn't an issue, current studies are underway to figure out why it appears the BBB in the typical obese person isn't letting them through. Hopefully the future will bring a greater understanding of how this complex system works and new interventions to help those suffering with weight issues.

In the meantime there are things we can do and other metabolic issues we can deal with (such as insulin resistance) to increase the likelihood of successful weight loss.

18 Andrea G. Izquierdo, Ana B. Crujeiras, Felipe F. Casanueva, Marcos C. Carreira. Leptin, Obesity, and Leptin *Resistance: Where Are We 25 Years Later? Nutrients.* 2019 Nov; 11(11): 2704. Published online 2019 Nov 8. doi: 10.3390/nu11112704. Retrieved from https://www.ncbi.nlm.nih.gov/pmc/articles/PMC6893721/ on 2022/02/08

19 Author: Taylor Evans, PHD candidate. *How Pathogens Penetrate the Blood-Brain Barrier. Published on The American Society for Microbiology* website on 2020/04/17. Retrieved from https://asm.org/Articles/2020/April/How-Pathogens-Penetrate-the-Blood-Brain-Barrier#:~:text=The%20blood%2Dbrain%20barrier%20is,direct%20contact%20with%20brain%20tissue.&text=The%20BBB%20is%20a%20compound,Endothelial%20Cells on 2022/03/08

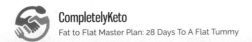

Toxins

We are surrounded by toxins. They are in our air, our food and in the water we drink every day. Many toxins are in our homes and in the places where we work. We absorb toxins from our environment as we go about daily activities and also as we sleep through the night. These toxins get into our bodies and build up in the liver and throughout the digestive system. I see this regularly in the group of clients who are doing everything right and yet are still struggling to lose those unwanted pounds. But this can be changed by:

- Cleaning up the environment as much as possible

- Employing strategies to detoxify the body

- Eating healthy food to nourish the gut biome and support liver function

When toxins build up in the gut they can cause gas and bloating, constant acid reflux (GERD), constipation or diarrhea, IBS and a leaky gut which leads to inflammation throughout the body. When the body has to deal with inflammation, weight loss slows down or can halt altogether.

Toxins in the environment

It's time to think about the products you purchase and bring into your home. When purchasing cleaning products, look for the ones that are unscented and bio-degradable. Laundry detergents should be the same and do you really need those chemical laden dryer sheets? The soaps you use on your body should be as pure as possible and also unscented; the same with shampoos, conditioners, make up and shaving creams.

Be aware of what you are buying and bringing into your home environment. Take time to inform yourself about the chemicals that are most harmful and in common use; read labels and avoid them! Take a walk through your home with possible toxin sources in mind and take action when you see the areas that need attention.

The air you breathe day in and day out could easily contain toxins. If you live in a recently constructed or renovated home this will undoubtedly be true. If your office is in a sealed building you will also be affected by some toxins floating around in the recycled air. Consider buying and using a good quality, portable air filter. And speaking of filters, make sure to attend to cleaning that furnace filter on a regular basis. Get the air ducts vacuumed out too. Also check the air conditioner and be meticulous about keeping it clean.

A good clean source of drinking water is important too. If you are able, consider installing a filter directly on the water line that comes into your house. If you can't do this, buy a water container that filters small amounts of water at a time. I have this type of water jug on my kitchen counter at all times, in full view. It gives me that needed visual cue to drink a glass, and the water I drink daily is always freshly filtered! If you live rurally and your water source is a well, make sure to get the water tested yearly and have the well flushed and scrubbed every few years.

When shopping for groceries buy organic foods, if you can. I know it's more expensive but your health is worth it. Just do the best you can on this front and always give the foods you eat a good wash before preparation.

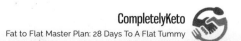

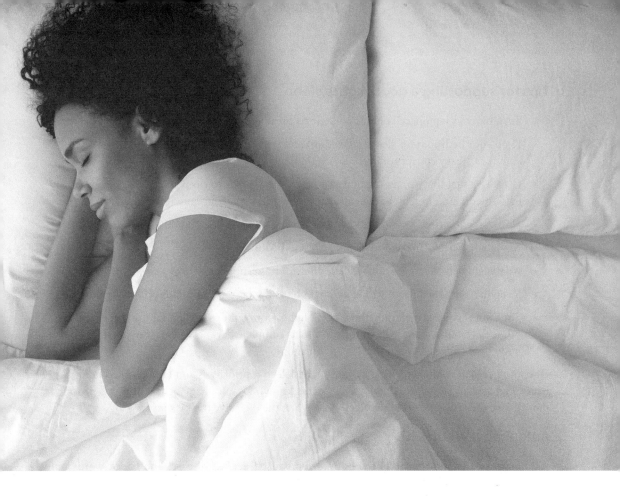

Sleep and weight loss

I can't stress the importance of a good night's sleep enough. There's plenty of evidence linking poor sleep habits to weight gain and unsuccessful weight loss. I recommend 7-9 hours of sleep each night to all of my clients. Here's why; a good night's sleep consistently could be a game-changer. A 2012 study looked at the relationship between sleep quality, quantity and weight loss in 245 women participating in a weight-loss intervention trial. This study showed women who reported getting 7 hours of sleep/night had "33% more likelihood of successful weight-loss" than the other group, who reported sleeping less than 7 hours/night over a 24 month period.[20] This is just one of many, many studies!

When you are tired your brain looks for rewards and is way more likely to focus on an immediate energy fix that comes in the form of indulging in carbohydrate laden snacks. We all know what happens then. Doing this on a regular basis will, at best, lead to a stall and at worst to weight gain.

Chronic lack of sleep also leads to chronic stress. The body releases cortisol when stressed. The release of cortisol into the bloodstream sends out a signal to slow down metabolism with the end result being that less calories get burned on a daily basis. No dieter wants this and if getting 7-9 hours of sleep each night is a way to impact cortisol levels, well then ... it's something worth working towards; more about cortisol later, in Chapter III: Dealing with Stress.

20 Thomson CA, Morrow KL, Flatt SW, Wertheim BC, Perfect MM, Ravia JJ, Sherwood NE, Karanja N, Rock CL. *Relationship between sleep quality and quantity and weight loss in women participating in a weight-loss intervention trial. Obesity (Silver Spring).* 2012 Jul;20(7):1419-25. doi: 10.1038/oby.2012.62. Epub 2012 Mar 8. PMID: 22402738; PMCID: PMC4861065. Retrieved from https://pubmed.ncbi.nlm.nih.gov/22402738/ on 2022/03/11

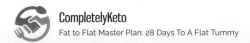

Tips for supporting a good night's sleep...

- Turn off your laptop, cell phone, and television at least an hour before bedtime.
- Keep your bedroom for sleep (relaxation) and release (sex) as opposed to work related activities, heavy conversations or entertainment.
- Create a ritual that signals the brain you are getting ready to sleep such as taking a warm bath, meditation or a bit of recreational (not work or study oriented) reading .
- Have a regular time for going to bed and getting up and adhere to this schedule every day.
- Avoid large, heavy meals and alcohol close to bedtime.
- No caffeinated beverages or chocolate after mid-afternoon.
- Sleep in a darkened room with good, light blocking curtains or blinds on the windows.
- Turn out the lights including those small lights from laptops, cell phones, alarm clocks or other electronics that are in your bedroom as complete darkness sends the signal for your body to release melatonin (the "sleep" hormone).

One more reason to make getting a good night's sleep a priority is something called autophagy. Every night when you sleep a biological process known as autophagy occurs and this process is more active towards the end of the sleep cycle when the digestive tract is empty.

Autophagy: What is it?

Autophagy is an important way the body defends itself against disease. The Greek words *auto* meaning self and *phagy* meaning eating is combined in the word autophagy; it literally means self-eating! This word perfectly describes the self-cannibalizing mechanism our body cells use to do housecleaning. By literally "eating up" oxidized particles, damaged proteins and broken cell bits during the autophagy process, our cells become unclogged and are better able to regenerate into healthy newer cells. A good night's sleep is essential for autophagy.

The process of autophagy is easily disrupted when the body is busy digesting food. It takes about 11 hours to digest food that's been ingested. A complete break from ingesting food supports autophagy, your body's natural process for house cleaning. That is why the process of autophagy occurs and is more active towards the end of the sleep cycle when the digestive tract is empty. [21] This is one more reason to make getting a good night's sleep a priority (and why pizza at midnight is never a good idea)!

Every night when we sleep one could say we are also fasting. Sleep is the time when the task of digesting food slows down. There are many benefits to lengthening the time we are not ingesting food into longer periods of fasting.

The take-away lesson learned from the rapid weight-loss bariatric surgery patients enjoy in the months immediately after their surgery is: fasting works for weight-loss. Of course, people who have had this surgery literally can't eat post-surgery and only slowly heal enough so that for quite a few months only very small amounts of food can be ingested. The result is rapid weight-loss. However while this surgery can be life-saving for some, for most of us battling the bulge it's a drastic solution.

21 Chauhan AK, Mallick BN. *Association between autophagy and rapid eye movement sleep loss-associated neurodegenerative and patho-physio-behavioral changes* Retrieved abstract from https://pubmed.ncbi.nlm.nih.gov/31605901/on 2022/03/09

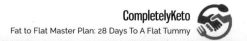
CompletelyKeto
Fat to Flat Master Plan: 28 Days To A Flat Tummy

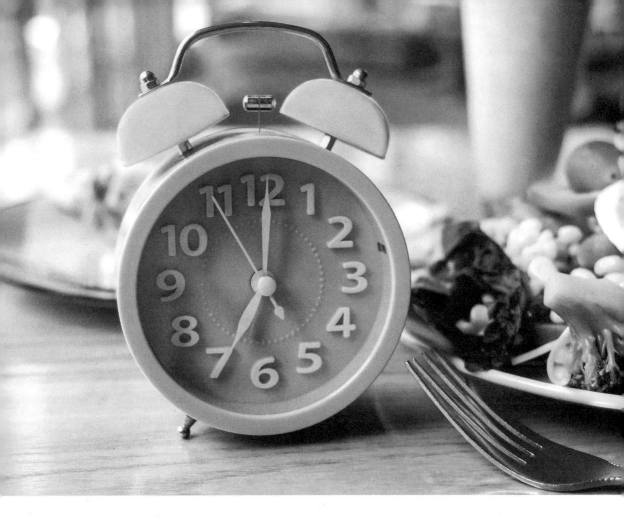

Intermittent Fasting (IF)

I believe a ketogenic approach to eating integrated with a program of *intermittent fasting* will not only kick start weight-loss for those just getting started but will also help break through a stubborn plateau. I have seen first-hand how the keto lifestyle when combine with intermittent fasting (IF) can actually reverse pre- diabetes, insulin resistance and even full-blown Type 2 diabetes for some of my clients.

Having said this we also have to stress the importance of consulting your physician before embarking on any new eating plan, including the one we are outlining in this book. Careful monitoring by your doctor will be necessary for anyone with diagnosed a medical condition(s).

Many of us are eating every two or three hours all day long. If our bodies are constantly in the process of digesting and processing the last ingestion of food when can they possibly switch over to using fat, stored in adipose tissue for energy? The short answer is they can't and they won't. The liver will be tied up all day processing glucose and guess what? Any extra will be converted to fat molecules and shipped off with the aid of insulin for storage as new body fat.

Eating three meals a day plus three or four snacks isn't working as a strategy for maintaining a healthy weight and body. You need at least 3 hours between meals to get insulin levels to drop. This is a key bit of information for the prevention of obesity. It is simple; longer gaps where no food is ingested drops insulin. This prevents high blood sugar and obesity. If you keep eating every hour or so, insulin never has a chance to drop and your blood sugar remains high, promoting obesity.

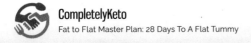

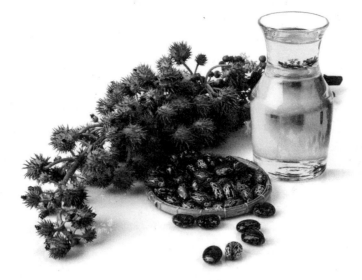

Simply defined, intermittent fasting describes periods of fasting interspersed with periods of eating normally. The length of the fasting periods and eating periods can vary. In his book, The Complete Guide to Fasting, Dr. Fung categorizes fasting periods as: "short, (less than 24 hours) or long, (more than 24 hours)." [22] A person undertaking a short fast will still be eating at least once a day. It isn't as hard as it sounds and works well for ongoing and sustained weight loss. Don't worry, I will only ask you to do this longer, 24 hour fast, once a week!

There are two types of intermittent fasts employed on the Fat to Flat Master Plan Program and both are short-term fasts:

- 12 hour fast: This is the usual over-night fast that happens every night. We break this fast in the morning with breakfast. If you finished your supper at 7:00 p.m. and ate breakfast the next morning the time in between these meals would be 12 hours; no bed-time snack and no refrigerator raids at midnight! You will be doing this every day to regulate insulin levels so your body can actually burn fat for energy.

- 24 hour fast: Also referred to as one meal a day or OMAD. Using the supper over at 7:00 p.m. model, a person practicing OMAD would skip both breakfast and lunch the next day and eat only the evening meal at 7:00 p.m.

Castor oil cleanse

Castor oil is made by pressing the oil out of Castor beans. These beans are actually seeds from the Ricinus communis plant. The oil is heated during the production process which deactivates the poisonous enzyme ricin, contained in the seeds. The end result is medicinal grade castor oil.

"The main chemical that exerts castor oil's laxative property is ricinoleic acid. In the intestine, lipase breaks down castor oil into ricinoleic acid, which activates EP3 and EP4 prostanoid receptors in smooth muscle cells. The activation of these receptors creates a transient calcium surge, which creates propulsion in the intestine. Due to this mechanism of action, castor oil falls in the stimulant laxative category ... " [23]

It's best to do this cleanse on a day when you don't have to go to work and are expecting no visitors. I suggest doing it on the first day that you begin this Fat to Flat Master Plan Program. That will be on a Sunday.

22 Fung, Jason MD & Moore, Jimmy. *The Complete Guide to Fasting: Heal Your Body Through Intermittent, Alternate-day and Extended Fasting*, ISBN 13: 978-1-628600-01-8,Victory Belt Publishing Inc., p.199

23 Aloukaran J, Tripp J. *Castor Oil*. [Updated 2021 Nov 24]. In: StatPearls [Internet]. Treasure Island (FL): StatPearls Publishing; 2022 Jan-. Retrieved from https://www.ncbi.nlm.nih.gov/books/NBK551626/ on 2022/03/05.

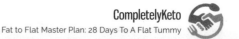

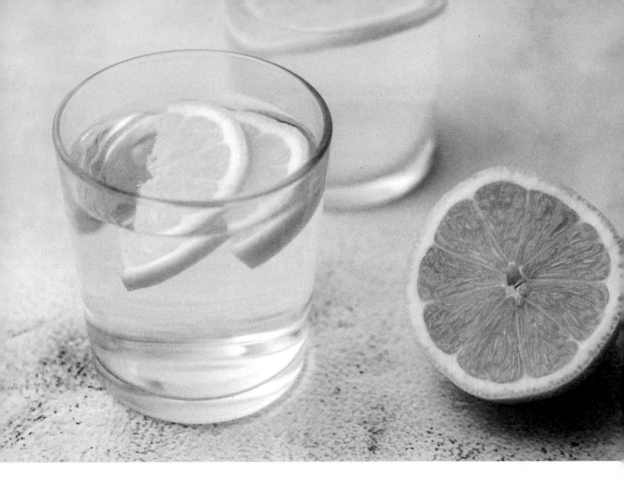

Castor Oil Cleanse recipe:

- 3 T medical grade castor oil
- 1/3 C freshly squeezed lemon juice
- 2/3 C water
- Small amount of stevia, to taste

Instructions:

1. Mix castor oil into the freshly squeezed lemon juice and add water. Stir in stevia, to taste. Drink this early in the morning on an empty stomach. Drink quickly, all at once.

2. Wait for ½ hour and drink 1 glass of hot water

3. Wait for 15 minutes and drink 2 more glasses of warm water.

4. Wait another 15 minutes and have 2 more glasses of warm water.

Relax until you need to go use the washroom. You will likely have 4-5 bowel movements in the next few hours. You may feel slightly light-headed as the flush is fairly intense and works as a detox which could also possibly flush out parasites that are sometimes present in the digestive tract.

Take it easy for the rest of the day and eat only a light meal in the evening; no fried or spicy foods. Do this flush no more than once every 6 months. While I highly recommend the castor oil cleanse at the beginning of the program it isn't mandatory; but you will have to choose between doing this detox on day #1 and practicing OMAD, a form of intermittent.

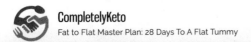

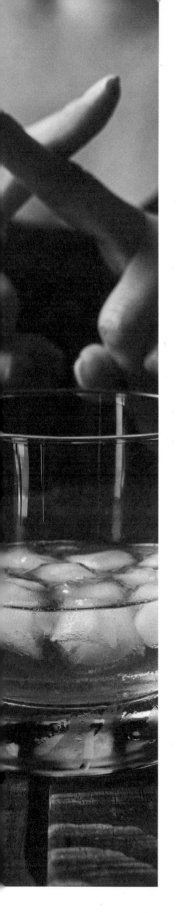

Day one fasting protocol

Fat to Flat Master Plan employs one day of OMAD a week. The first of these fasts occurs on day #1 of the program. For the following 3 weeks every Monday will be an OMAD day. OMAD is an acronym for one meal a day. It describes a form of intermittent fasting that embraces a menu plan based on twenty three hours of fasting with a one hour window for taking in food hence; one meal a day, OMAD.

When employed at the beginning of this program, OMAD provides your body the opportunity to use up its stored glycogen reserve and will help you get into ketosis faster. On this first day, your evening meal will be light and easy to digest. You will have a 60 minute window during the evening in which to consume this meal.

Drinks to avoid ...

The following drinks are not included in this month long program:

- Carbonated drinks: It's well-known that carbonated drinks can cause bloating and gas. For some this just means a bit of burping but for those dealing with acid reflux, GERD, IBS and other digestive issues the bloating can be very uncomfortable. As well, many carbonated diet drinks are loaded with artificial sweeteners that also cause disruption in the gut, so I simply recommend leaving them out of your menu plan.

- Drinks with ice: The normal core body temperature is 98.6 F. It takes energy to warm up the body's internal temperature after an ice cold drink. Ayurvedic medicine practitioners believe cold drinks slow down the digestion process and recommend against icing beverages. Western medicine is less concerned about this but a very small study from 2013 showed that athletes actually drank more cool water (rather than iced water or room temperature water) when given these options for re-hydrating after exercise.[24] The temperature of the water was 16 F, which is the average temperature of cool water, coming from the tap. While my preference is to drink water at room temperature I recommend that my clients drink water that is no lower than 16 F in temperature and never drink any beverages with added ice.

- Dairy (other than drinks made using full fat yogurt and kefir): This includes milk from cows, goats or soy. You may use a small amount of nut milk if allergic to dairy.

- Alcohol: Drinking alcohol won't necessarily kick you out of ketosis but there's no doubt it will slow ketosis down. Here's why. Your body deals with alcohol like it's a poison that it must get rid of right away. So, your liver will stop working on producing ketones from fat and will immediately focus on processing the alcohol.

24 Abdollah Hosseinlou, Saeed Khamnei, Masumeh Zamanlu. *The effect of water temperature and voluntary drinking on the post rehydration sweating.* Int J Clin Exp Med. 2013; 6(8): 683–687. Published online 2013 Sep 1. Retrieved from https://www.ncbi.nlm.nih.gov/pmc/articles/PMC3762624/ on 2022/03/05

 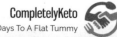

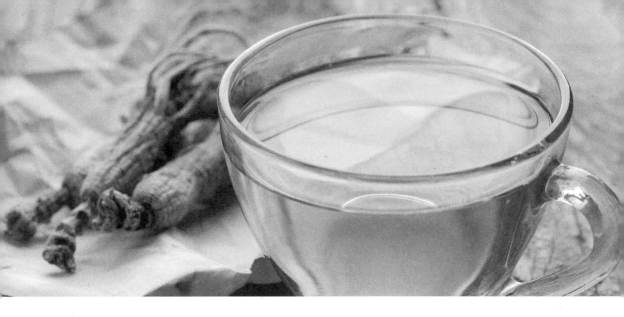

Drinks to be included daily ...

Here is a list of drinks I want you to include on a daily basis while following the Fat to Flat Master Plan program:

- Anti-inflammatory Drink: I want you to enjoy this Anti-inflammatory Drink first thing every morning. The ingredients are easy to find and have all been selected for their ability to lessen inflammation in the body.

- 5 cups of herbal tea daily: Herbal teas have been selected that boost your metabolism and/or soothe the digestive tract and aid in detoxifying the body. You should rotate the teas you select daily. I will provide the time of day for drinking the following teas in your daily menu plan:

  1. Green Tea with Ginger

  2. Tangerine Peel Tea

  3. Ginseng Tea

  4. Oolong tea

  5. Banyan Detox Digest Tea

- Bedtime Triphala Drink: Used for thousands of years in Ayurvedic medicine practice, Triphala is beneficial for digestion and elimination. It acts as a mild laxative and digestive tonic, stabilizes blood sugar and provides a good source of antioxidants and vitamin C. I recommend taking the powdered form of triphala in a Triphala Bedtime Drink, every evening.

- Metabolic Blast drinks: Not only do infused waters encourage you to drink more to stay well hydrated because of their superb flavors they also have many health benefits and energy boosting properties depending on what you use to make them. I encourage you to make both hot and cold drinks infused with your favorite spices, fruits and veggies. Here's a few of my own concoctions that are provided in my list of Basic Recipes:

- Lemon Ginger Water

- Berry Blast Water

- Cinnamon/Anise Tea

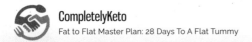

Chapter II: Dealing with Stress

Cortisol Factor

Your body has a natural response that kicks in automatically when you encounter a threat. An area at the base of the brain, springs into action and sends various signals (through nerve and hormonal systems) that work to stimulate the adrenal glands which are located on top of the kidneys. The adrenal glands release adrenaline and cortisol. If you've ever experienced a sudden fright you know what a surge of adrenalin and cortisol does to your body as it goes into a state of high alert; your heart pounds, you sweat profusely and your thoughts sharpen as you prepare to deal with whatever threatens.

Adrenalin works to:

- raise blood pressure
- increase heart rate
- increase glucose supply in the blood for the needed burst of energy

Cortisol works to:

- increase glucose in the bloodstream
- increase the release of substances that work to repair bodily tissues
- enhance the brain's ability to process and use glucose

The cortisol release also works to slow down or completely stop unnecessary bodily functions that would impair a quick response to the perceived threat. This includes:

- alteration of the immune system response
- suppression of normal digestion activity
- suppression of the reproductive system
- suppression of growth[25]

This state of high alert is meant to be temporary and once hormone levels return to normal, blood pressure goes down, heart rate slows, your body relaxes and bodily functions should normalize and resume. But here's the thing; many of us are in a state of constant stress; juggling family life, work expectations and difficult relationships, etc. The list is long and ever-changing. We often are bombarded with stressful situations on a daily basis and the resulting cortisol response in particular, leaves us vulnerable to many health problems, including:

---

25 Author: Mayo Clinic Staff. *Chronic Stress puts your Health at Risk*. Retrieved from https://www.mayoclinic.org/healthy-lifestyle/stress-management/in-depth/stress/art-20046037#:~:text=Cortisol%2C%20the%20primary%20stress%20hormone,fight%2Dor%2Dflight%20situation. On 2022/03/07

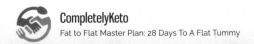

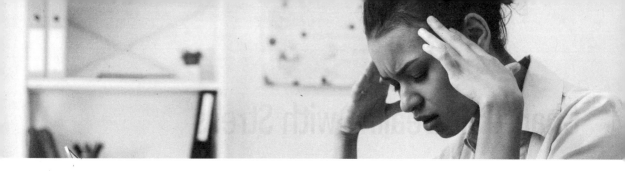

- mental health issues (anxiety, depression, foggy thinking)

- compulsive eating, weight gain, weight loss stalls

- poor digestion

- sleeplessness

- high blood pressure, heart attack and stroke

This list could be much longer but you get the idea. Constant stress affects your health and consequently, your quality of life. We all need to find ways to lessen daily stress.

Quick test for checking cortisol levels

I counsel my clients to do a quick test to check their cortisol levels at the beginning of the Fat to Flat Master Plan program. It is optional but highly recommended especially if you are experiencing:

- persistent fatigue

- headaches

- foggy thinking and difficulty with concentration

- weight gain or loss (with no behavioral explanations)

- muscle weakness

- high blood pressure

- irritability

- low blood sugar

These symptoms could be indicating either high or low cortisol levels. I suggest a test which works using easy-to-collect saliva and provides for testing cortisol levels in the morning, at noon, in the early evening and late evening. This test kit, for at home use, can be purchased online if not available at your local pharmacy. Once the specimens are collected you mail them to an accredited lab that sends you the results through the mail.

Meditation for stress relief ...

Stress in daily life is pretty much a given so it's important to develop some strategies for coping. Stress can be managed and finding appropriate coping mechanisms is important for your weight-loss goals and overall well-being.

Meditation helps to clear the mind of all the needless thoughts that create stress. By focusing attention on one particular object, an image or reciting a mantra, meditation can induce a state of calmness which helps the whole body achieve greater health and well-being. Meditation is a practice that can be performed anywhere. It can be performed while sitting, standing or lying down. Some of these practices can be used while walking, riding the bus or even while at work or school.

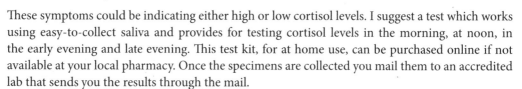

CompletelyKeto
Fat to Flat Master Plan: 28 Days To A Flat Tummy

Here are three, easy to learn and implement meditation techniques:

1. Guided meditation: Sometimes called guided imagery or visualization, with this method of meditation you form mental images of places or situations you find relaxing. You try to use as many senses as possible, such as smells, sights, sounds and textures. You may be led through this process by a guide or teacher. Guided meditations are easily found on YouTube and various online websites. Numerous apps are also available for purchase.

2. Mantra meditation: In this type of meditation, you silently repeat a calming word, thought or phrase to prevent distracting thoughts.

3. Mindfulness meditation: This type of meditation is based on being mindful, or having an increased awareness and acceptance of living in the present moment. In mindfulness meditation, you broaden your conscious awareness. You focus on what you experience during meditation, such as the flow of your breath. You can observe your thoughts and emotions, but let them pass without judgment.

Breathing exercises for daily stress relief...

Often stressful situations arise quickly. Four breathing techniques, that can lower your stress level in a matter of minutes, are outlined below:

1. Change your breathing pattern: Focus on the breath and simply change the way you are breathing. Use this strategy anywhere. You could be in a subway or a meeting at work and no-one around you will be the wiser:

2. Breathe in through your nose as you notice the air going deep into your belly. Count to three as you inhale slowly; hold for one second then exhale slowly, through your nose, on a count of three.

3. Imagine you are breathing in peaceful, calming energy and exhaling tension and stress.

4. Count backwards while breathing slowly: Count backwards slowly, starting at 10, taking one complete breath (inhale and exhale) on each count. By the time you reach zero you will likely feel calmer or more relaxed. Repeat if you feel like you need another round, from 10 to 0.

5. Sitting Exercise: This one takes slightly more time but can still be done quickly. It's a great way to take a mini break as well as working to reduce stress. While sitting with legs and ankles uncrossed, mentally check your facial muscles and consciously relax any tension; let your jaw drop slightly and relax the muscles in your forehead and jaw. Allow both arms to fall gently by your sides as your shoulders lower slightly. Let hands dangle and release any tension in fingers. Imagine that your feet are growing roots deep beneath the surface while being aware of how your thighs and buttocks feel against the surface where you sit. Now breath as you would for exercise #1.

6. 4/7/8 Breath: This is a repeated breathing exercise for relaxation; to be employed twice a day. Sit in a straight backed chair with your feet flat on the floor. Let your tongue rest gently on the roof of your mouth with its tip just behind the ridge at the back of your upper teeth. Breathe in through your nose to a count of four, hold for a count of seven then exhale through your mouth to a count of eight while making a whoosh sound. This is one cycle. Repeat three more times. Develop the habit of doing this at least twice a day.

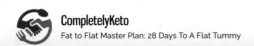

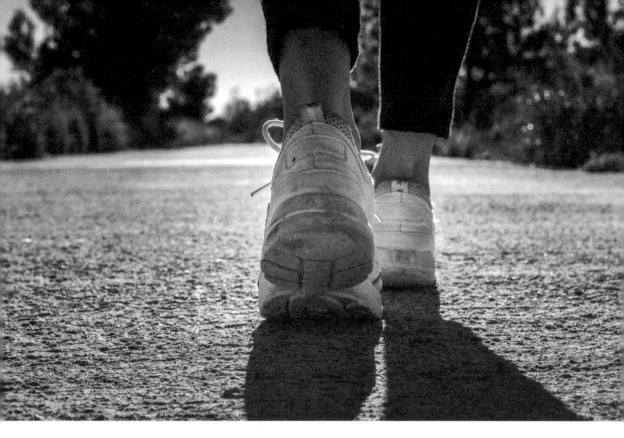

Therapy

Some of my clients have benefited from various forms of professional counseling or therapy. The behaviors that literally fuel weight gain are often due to coping mechanisms, developed early in life. Many therapists are trained to deal with past traumatic experiences, depression and other issues that often affect weight-loss efforts. I urge everyone that is struggling with their eating program and weight-loss attempts to consider engaging professional counsel. A therapist can help you unravel the hidden blocks that are holding you back and will provide support as you develop new ways of being in the world. Your health care provider should be able to refer you to an appropriate specialist in your area.

30 minute brisk walk daily ...

I recommend the activity of walking for my clients in most of my programs. This exercise works to burn up stores of glycogen at the beginning of a keto diet but I also encourage my clients to continue the walking routine beyond the transition period. Walking is recommended for 30 minutes every day, first thing in the morning. I want you to burn off any glucose that's accumulated in the form of glycogen so your body will start producing ketones for energy as early in the day as possible. Once the body's store of glucose is used up during a 30 minute morning walk you will then switch to burning stored body fat for energy.

A brisk walk will quickly boost endorphin levels in your brain. Getting outside and away from the sources of stress provides immediate relief. A 2018 study confirms that being outside closer to nature in a wilderness setting relieves both physical and psychological stress.[26] The effects are measureable, so scheduling time to walk outside in a close by park or nature reserve (if possible) will be a pleasurable antidote to the pressures of everyday living.

---

26 Ewart, Alan and Chang, Yun. *Levels of nature and stress response.* Retrieved from https://www.mdpi.com/2076-328X/8/5/49 on 2/5/21

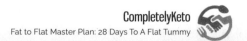

CompletelyKeto

Fat to Flat Master Plan: 28 Days To A Flat Tummy

Chapter III: Supplementation

Support your body ...

If you've been following one of my other ketogenic food plans you will already be familiar with my recommended list of supplements. It's important to take the list of supplements that follows seriously. If you do and you add these supplements to your daily regimen you will greatly enhance the weight loss success you achieve during this month.

Electrolytes

An electrolyte is a chemical that is capable of conducting electricity when mixed with water. Electrolytes necessary for normal bodily functions include:

- Sodium
- Potassium
- Calcium
- Bicarbonate
- Magnesium
- Chloride
- Phosphate

Here's an example ... muscles use calcium, sodium, and potassium when they contract. Each time your heart beats it's actually contracting in a specific rhythm. If electrolytes become too imbalanced, it can lead to weakness in muscles. Excessive contraction (as in muscle cramps) can also occur. It's easy to deduce that where the heart is concerned; we need electrolytes to survive and we need them in the proper proportions.

Leg cramps are common during or after a work-out and athletes often replenish electrolytes lost through sweat by having an electrolyte drink after exertion. While it's good to take in electrolytes when depletion is suspected it's important to read labels as electrolyte drinks are often full of hidden sugars.

One of the reasons we encourage hydrating by drinking chicken (and other bone broths) on the Fat to Flat Master Plan program is to naturally supplement the body with certain electrolytes. The long slow simmering process involved in making bone stocks of all kinds leeches electrolytes like calcium, phosphate and sodium from nutrient dense bones that often go to waste. You are encouraged to take a cup of bone broth whenever you feel the need during the Extreme Speed Keto process.

Sodium

Drinking water and specific teas at regular intervals during the day is extremely important during Fat to Flat Master Plan. In fact you will probably need to find ways of reminding yourself to take in another sip of H2O. Keeping a water container close by will quickly become a habit.

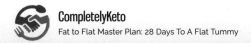

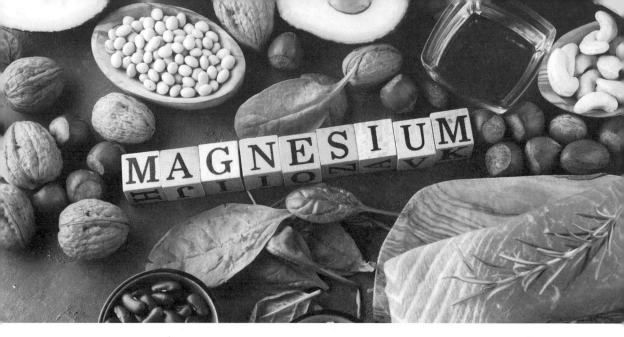

But along with drinking more water and following a ketogenic diet comes a need to urinate more often and with that there may be a need for more sodium. This may be especially true since you will have eliminated all that excess salt from packaged foods and much of your daily intake will come from the sodium you add to your meals in the form of salt.

When selecting a salt look for either sea salt or rock salt. We are particularly fond of the pink Himalayan salt that can be found in most supermarkets today. Both sea salt and rock salt will add other important minerals to your daily diet.

Potassium can also be depleted just like sodium due to the diuretic effect that is part of any diet low in carbohydrate content. Your tasty bone broth will help add the much needed sodium and potassium to your daily intake.

This brings us to magnesium because it's needed in order for your body to be able to absorb potassium properly. Often potassium levels are low in the body because there is an insufficient level of magnesium present.

Magnesium

While there will be magnesium present in your broth it may not be in a high enough quantity to give you what you need each day. Most people are deficient in magnesium from the get go. This is true for a number of reasons:

- For city dwellers the available drinking water goes through a filtering process which ends up removing most of its magnesium content; the same is true for bottled waters
- The process of "softening" water removes magnesium
- While magnesium is present in some foods it is not there in sufficient quantities making it hard to take in adequate magnesium through diet alone

While on the Fat to Flat Master Plan program it is recommended that you take 400-800 milligrams of magnesium daily. There are different types of magnesium available on drugstore and health food shop shelves but we recommend taking magnesium glycinate because it is easier for the body to absorb in this form.

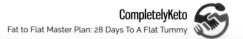

Magnesium can cause loose stools for some people. If this is the case then split your daily dose up, taking 400 milligrams in the morning with food and another 400 at lunchtime; again with food. If this dosage still proves to be too much then switch to taking a smaller dose each time.

Cramping muscles can also be soothed by a good soak in a warm tub with a few cups of Epsom salts added in as the bath water is running.

If you have any concerns at all, be sure to consult with your family doctor.

Vitamin D

Exposure to the sun is by far the best (and most economical) way to raise vitamin D levels in the body. Many North Americans are deficient in Vitamin D. Those living the farthest distance from the equator are the ones most likely to be afflicted. Today we all wear brimmed hats and protective clothes in an effort to protect our eyes and skin from UV rays; this, along with sunscreens that are lathered on liberally further complicate the problem.

According to a WebMD article: "Exposure of the hands, face, arms, and legs to sunlight two to three times a week for about one-fourth of the time it would take to develop a mild sunburn will cause the skin to produce enough vitamin D." [27]

If you don't get enough time in the sun then it may be prudent to take a vitamin D supplement. Correct dosages vary according to body weight and current vitamin D levels in the body.

Full spectrum enzymes

Enzymes work to speed up chemical reactions and many chemical reactions in your body are regulated by enzymes. They work to catalyze the pathways of cell metabolism including the digestion of large molecules like carbohydrates, proteins and fats. Enzymes assist with breaking them down into smaller more easily absorbed molecules:

- Simple sugars (glucose) from carbohydrates
- Amino acids from protein
- Cholesterol from fats

Many of these digestive enzymes are produced by the pancreas and intestines as well as in the salivary glands and stomach. It's possible to have a healthy diet yet be deficient in nutrients if digestive enzymes are not present in high enough quantity.

Enzyme deficiency can be caused by certain diseases as well as inflammation in the digestive tract. Food allergies and sensitivities, IBS, diverticulitis, leaky gut, aging, low stomach acid and stress are only a few of the things that could contribute to insufficient digestive enzymes with chronic stress being a major contributor.

Finding ways to reduce stress and eating a healthy balanced diet can help restore normal digestion but sometimes supplementation with digestive enzymes is beneficial.

---

27 WebMD website. Article title: *Vitamin D*. Retrieved from https://www.webmd.com/vitamins/ai/ingredientmono-929/vitamin-d on 20/05/2018.

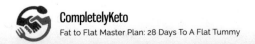

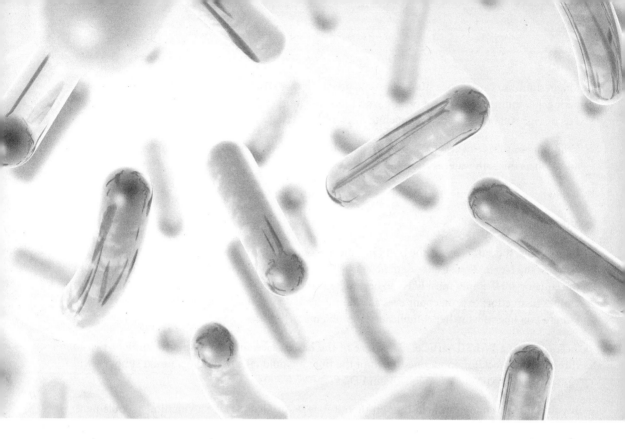

If you choose to supplement with digestive enzymes choose a product that includes a variety of enzymes. Read the label and look for a product that includes:

- proteases for breaking down proteins
- lipases for breaking down fats
- carbohydrases (amylase) for breaking down carbohydrates

Probiotics

Inside the digestive tract we have trillions of bacteria. We call this micro-biome "gut flora". A healthy and functioning gut flora:

- helps in the digestion of food
- assists in detoxifying harmful compounds
- produces vitamins as well as other nutrients
- balances the immune system

These good bacteria can be decimated when antibiotics are introduced. They are wiped out along with the bad bacteria that the antibiotic is actually targeting. This, along with chronic stress, is one of the biggest culprits for disrupting a healthy gut flora population.

Probiotics can be taken to restore gut flora and come in powdered form, usually in a capsule. The last 10 years have seen an uptick on understanding gut health and its importance for over-all health but there are still many questions that need answering. Research is ongoing.

If you decide to take a probiotic look for a reputable brand that includes both Lactobacillus and *Bifidobacterium*.

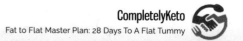

CompletelyKeto

Fat to Flat Master Plan: 28 Days To A Flat Tummy

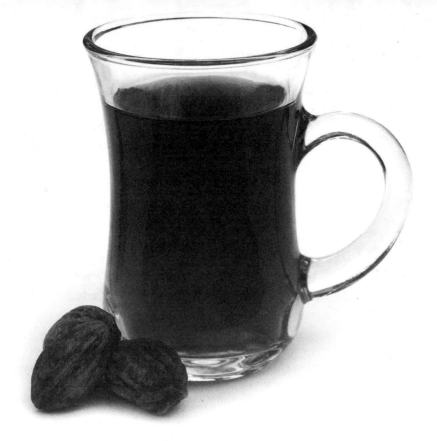

Triphala

Triphala is an Ayurvedic herbal powder made from three fruits:

- Amalaki (or Indian Gooseberry): Full of antioxidants, Indian gooseberry helps to remove toxins from the body. It will help bolster the health of the pancreas, aids in the regulation of cholesterol levels and works to keep your bones strong.

- Bibhitaki (also known as black myrobalan): Bibhitaki also helps regulate cholesterol levels and works on keeping muscle as well as bones, healthy and strong.

- Haritaki: This fruit, which has a nut-like appearance, is an excellent antiflammatory as well as an antioxidant.

Used for thousands of years in Ayurvedic medicine practice, Triphala is beneficial for digestion and elimination. It acts as a mild laxative and digestive tonic, stabilizes blood sugar and provides a good source of antioxidants and vitamin C.

I recommend taking the powdered form of triphala in a bedtime drink, every night. The powder has a somewhat bitter flavor so my drink recipe includes stevia and a bit of lime or lemon juice to mask the astringent taste.

Bedtime Triphala Drink Recipe

- Stir 1 tsp of triphala into ½ C of warm water

- Add 1 T of lemon or lime juice

- Sweeten with liquid or powdered stevia, to taste.

I purchase this brand of triphala online.

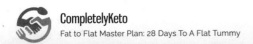

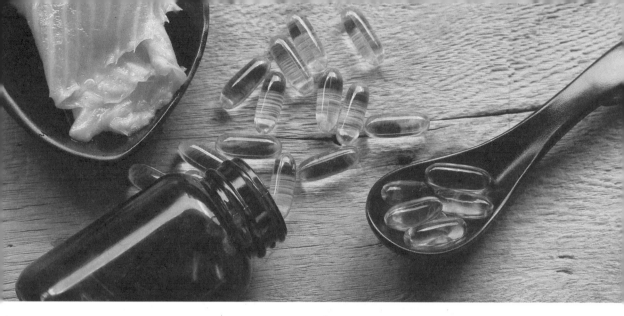

Fish oil

As discussed earlier the typical western diet with poor meat quality, fast foods, processed foods and vegetable oils lacks Omega-3 fatty acids (EPA and DHA) and is overly rich in pro-inflammatory omega-6 fatty acids. For many people the resulting systemic inflammation causes a wide range of negative health consequences.

Your body cannot make EPA or DHA and you must get them from the foods you eat or from supplementation. Fish oil is a potent source of these anti-inflammatory fatty acids and is also readily available in liquid or capsule form.

Fish oil will affect the "stickiness" of platelets so you should consult your physician if you have any bleeding issues, are taking blood thinners or have a surgery scheduled in the near future.

Krill oil

Krill oil is an extract prepared from a tiny crustacean, Euphausia Superb, which is a species of Antarctic krill. It contains similar omega-3 fatty acids to fish oil but usually has higher levels of EPA.

Krill oil omega-3s are attached to phospholipids, which make them more easily absorbed by the body than the triglyceride form of omega-3s found in fish oil.

Since the source for krill oil is a crustacean anyone with an allergy to shell-fish should exercise caution if considering taking this supplement.

Bentonite clay

Clay is found in deposits all over the world. The clay that is used for health related interventions results from the natural process of volcanic ash aging over many, many years (from ancient volcanoes). It is also found in sedimentation basins. I prefer a type of clay found here in the United States in the area surrounding Fort Benton, Wyoming, hence the name; bentonite clay. There are two types of bentonite clay: Calcium bentonite clay and sodium bentonite clay. Sodium bentonite clay is used for industrial applications and calcium bentonite clay has more medical uses. Bentonite clay is an ancient treatment that has a long history of medicinal uses. The numerous benefits of calcium bentonite clay can be accessed two ways.

 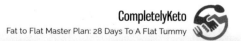

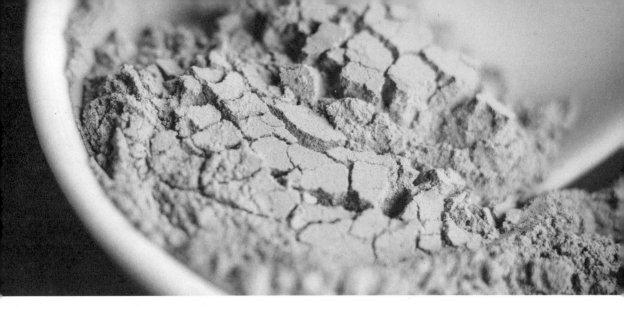

- Application of a clay poultice: The clay poultice is believed to effectively draw various toxins, out through the skin. Due to its negative charge the clay attracts and then absorbs toxins (that have a positive charge) from the body.

- Ingesting a calcium bentonite clay drink: Make a drink with 1 tsp human grade (edible) calcium bentonite clay mixed into 6-8 oz of filtered (purified) water. Now when you stir the clay it water give it five minutes to settle. You want to drink the water but leave the clay on the bottom. You can have this drink once a day (optional)

For my clients embarking on the Fat to Flat Master Plan program I suggest using a calcium bentonite clay poultice on the abdomen, sometime during the week-end before starting the program. When selecting a bentonite clay for purchase be sure to get the calcium bentonite clay that's labeled edible and certified for human use. You can also use green clay for the poultice but bentonite clay is preferred.

To make a wet clay place powdered clay in a mixing bowl. Add a small amount of room temperature filtered water and mix it into the clay powder using a wooden or plastic spoon (do NOT use a metal bowl or spoon). Keep adding water and stirring the mixture until it reaches a consistency that is similar to that of peanut butter. Spread this clay onto a piece of cloth cut to a size that will fit over the area you want to treat, in this case your abdomen. I use muslin but a few layers of cheesecloth also work well. If you haven't made enough wet clay just repeat the process until you have a 1/8" thickness of clay spread across the fabric. Once the poultice is prepared follow these instructions:

- Lay the poultice directly on top of the skin across the abdomen allowing the clay itself to contact the skin directly.

- Use a skin-safe bandage tape to hold the poultice in place.

- Leave the poultice on until the clay is dry. Some choose to leave the poultice on overnight but, since only a thin layer of clay is used in this poultice, it won't take all night to dry.

- When the clay has dried, peel the cloth away and remove the clay from your skin. Use a damp cloth to remove any bits of dried clay left behind.

- Discard the used clay as it will be contaminated with the toxins removed from your body as the clay dried.

As always we recommend that everyone consult with their physician or primary health care provider before starting any new diet or program of supplementation

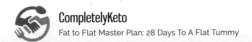

Chapter IV: Fermented Foods for Gut Health

What is fermentation?

Fermentation is a *living* process that utilizes a specific salt concentration to safely ferment vegetables without killing off the beneficial bacteria. During the fermentation process, the use of salty brine encourages beneficial bacteria to eat the sugars in the fermenting vegetables as they transform into pickles. Lacto-fermented pickles are cultured, and full of probiotics. They are not cooked, and can only be stored for long periods of time at low temperatures (as in a refrigerator or in a cooler root cellar area of the basement). Most people find that fermented vegetables have a mellow flavor as opposed to the sharper, tangy flavor of veggies put through the pickling process.

Some examples of fermented foods on the Fat to Flat Master Plan program are:

- Sauerkraut
- Kimchi
- A variety of fermented pickles
- Fermented salsa
- Fermented hot sauce
- Yogurt
- Kefir
- Tofu
- Tempeh
- Miso

What is pickling?

Most of us are more familiar with the pickling process. Pickling is a sterile process for preserving food. This means there are no living microorganisms involved in the pickling process. Instead, hot acidic liquid is utilized to sterilize and preserve vegetables. Sealing jarred vinegar pickles in a hot water bath is very common. Foods can also be canned under high pressure in a sealed pressure canner.

When we make pickles this way, we cook both the pickles and the brine. The result; these pickles can be stored at room temperature in their sealed jars for a long time without spoiling. Most pickles you purchase in a grocery store will have been prepared in this manner.

Finding fermented pickles and other fermented foods to purchase might take a bit more sleuthing; or you can make them at home. I've provided several recipes in Chapter VIII, so give it a try.

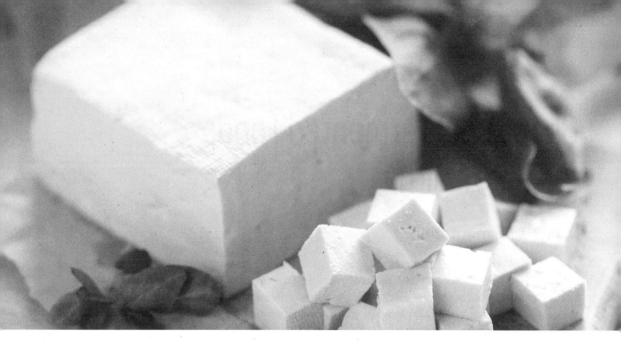

Fermented dairy products

Sensitivity to dairy is a common issue and often people aren't aware that their body isn't tolerating this food group. In the past I've found that limiting dairy works for a better weight loss outcome. If this is the case, taking the month away from eating dairy daily allows inflammation to lessen throughout the body and gives the gut a chance to heal. No doubt you are wondering why I am including some dairy products in this version of speed keto.

Many fermented dairy products are readily available at the supermarket or health food store. Even though only a very small amount of dairy is included in my other keto programs, I'm including these dairy products on the Fat to Flat Master Plan program for one good reason. Fermented dairy is full of probiotics that are proven to be of benefit to the gut microbiome. Including yogurt, kefir and even a small amount of aged cheese (occasionally) will add interesting variety to your menu and these foods are an abundant source of "good" bacteria.[28]

I've included recipes for two different types of homemade yogurt as well as kefir but if you elect to purchase commercial varieties of these products make sure to check their labels. You should only purchase products that are made with "live cultures". Also make there are no added sugars and opt for plain yogurt or kefir made with full fat dairy or coconut milk.

Fermented soy products: Tofu and tempeh

The same is true of fermented legume products like tofu and tempeh; only purchase products that contain "live culture". Tofu is actually made from soy milk that is fermented and made into blocks that vary in texture from silken (very soft) to soft as well as firm.

Tempeh differs in that it is made from whole soy beans that are fermented, and then pressed into firm blocks. It has a flavor that is unique and hard to describe; kind of earthy and nut-like. Tofu tends to be more neutral in taste and absorbs the other flavor profiles of ingredients in recipes where it is included. For this reason I often employ marinades when cooking with tofu.

28 Authosr: Daniel J. Lisko, G. Patricia Johnston, Carl G Johnston. Academic Editor: Giuseppe Comi. *Effects of Dietary Yogurt on the Healthy Human Gastrointestinal (GI) Microbiome. Microorganisms.* 2017 Mar; 5(1): 6. Published online 2017 Feb 15. doi: 10.3390/microorganisms5010006. Retrieved from https://www.ncbi.nlm.nih.gov/pmc/articles/PMC5374383/ on 2022/03/03

 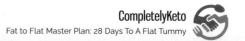

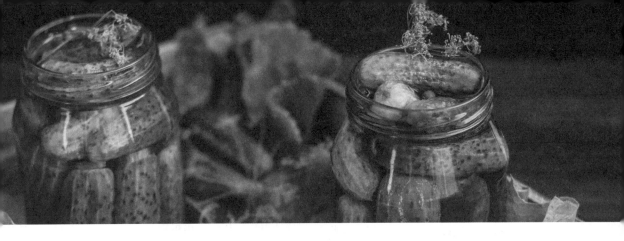

Using a culture to speed up fermentation

Lactobacilli are the primary genus of bacteria that work to convert sugar into lactic acid in fermented foods. Some foods can be successfully fermented through a process we call "wild fermentation" which simply means no cultures are added to aid the fermentation process. Lactobacilli are everywhere; i.e. on our skin, on countertops as well as on the outside of the vegetables we want to ferment. Given enough time this bacteria will work to eat up the naturally occurring sugars in these vegetables rendering them more acidic and producing the sourness we associate with the fermentation process.

Because this style of fermentation relies on only the bacteria naturally present and uses no added cultures we call the process, "wild fermentation". While most vegetables can be fermented this way a starter culture can be added anyway, to shorten the fermentation period. Cultures can be purchased for this use but here are a few suggestions you may already have on hand if you want to try to speed up the fermentation times for the recipes I've included in the program:

- Whey (the Liquid that separates out from homemade yogurt)
- The powder contained in a pro-biotic capsule
- Liquid from foods you have already fermented such as 1 or 2 T from home-made sauerkraut or fermented cucumber pickles ...

Some of my recipes will require longer fermentation periods without the addition of a culture. Since this is a month-long program you won't be able to use these fermented foods in your menu plan until the end of the month! Try adding the above cultures to see if you can speed up the fermentation process for earlier use. Even better; set up some jars of fermenting vegetables a week or two before you start the program!

What is a ferment weight?

A fermentation weight does exactly what the name implies; it will weigh down your vegetables during *fermentation*. This means it actually needs to have enough weight to hold food down inside the jar, beneath the brine. You also want a weight that can be easily cleaned after use. A non-porous material fits the bill, so my weight of choice is made from glass.

In a few of my recipes I've described a method of weighing veggies down by using the large folded outer leaves from cabbage. This method can be used successfully when making sauerkraut and kimchi but a glass fermentation weight would probably be more successful, simply because it has more weight. If you decide to make your own fermented veggies on a regular basis you may want to consider a fermentation weight purchase online.

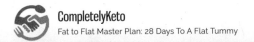

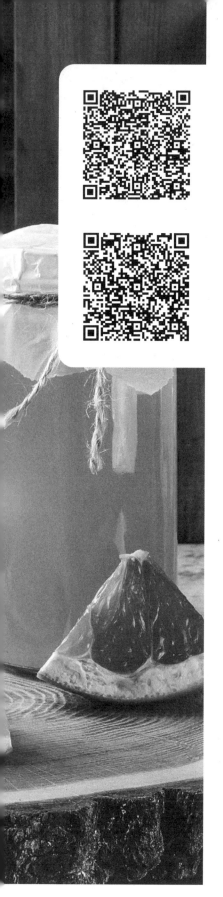

Here's where they can be found:

- MasonJarLifestyle.com
- Amazon.com

What is a fermenting lid?

A fermenting lid is made to fit on top of a wide mouthed mason jar. There are vents on top of these lids that will allow the naturally forming gases, created during the fermentation process, to escape. There are different styles readily available online here or here.

Most of you that are just starting to experiment with the fermenting process will not have fermenting lids on hand. Not to worry! You can use regular lids but will have to "burp" these jars daily to release air or gas pressure from the jar. If you are simply tying muslin or cheesecloth over-top the jar while fermenting, there will be no need for burping as air and gases can easily escape through the cloth.

Choose the right container ...

Foods that are being fermented should be placed in either glass jars or glazed ceramic crock containers. Never use plastic containers for fermenting veggies, even the plastics that are labeled "food safe". The acidic liquid produced during fermentation will leach compounds from the plastic you don't want to ingest.

Kombucha

Kombucha is a fermented tea drink made using a scoby or what many call the "Mother". The scoby is actually a symbiotic colony of yeast and bacteria. Kombucha has been around in Asia for at least 2,000 years. From there it spread in popularity through Russia and into Europe. More recently Kombucha has been appearing on our grocery shelves and is readily available at most supermarkets, health food stores and even in the cooler at the local gas station convenience store. While I highly recommend drinking kombucha, because it is so beneficial for gut health, it isn't required. Kombucha is a good source of B vitamins and is often consumed by people who struggle with digestive issues like constipation, diarrhea, and IBS. The lactic acid bacteria, present in kombucha is a probiotic that encourages the growth of the "good" bacteria needed in a healthy functioning micro-biome. Also considered a thermogenic drink, it is believed to boost energy levels and aid in weight-loss; both good reasons to add it to your daily menu plan.[29] There are many, sugar free versions available commercially. As always, read labels carefully before purchasing. Look for the no sugar, low carb versions of this healthy fermented drink.

29 Author: Matt Smith. Reviewed by: Brunilda Nazario, MD. Kombucha. Retieved from https://www.webmd.com/diet/the-truth-about-kombucha#091e9c5e815dcf37-1-4 on 2022/03/2022

CompletelyKeto
Fat to Flat Master Plan: 28 Days To A Flat Tummy

Chapter V: Allowed Foods

Select "Quality" Foods

Organic is best when selecting veggies and "in season", locally grown is also recommended. Choose pastured, grass fed meats, game meats and wild-caught fish and salmon. Free range poultry and eggs as well as organic oils should also top the shopping list.

I know that locally sourced and organically grown foods are more expensive but when your well-being and the health of your family is at stake, the quality of the foods you purchase really matters. If you are dealing with a tight budget then do the best you can, keeping in mind that there may be other places where you can trim monthly spending besides the weekly grocery bill.

Please note I have not made use of all the foods listed in this chapter when creating the meal plan and the recipes that go along with plan. You can substitute ingredients using only the food listed here. I want the meals you prepare to reflect your own personal preferences

Fats

At the turn of the last century in the early 1900's, butter and lard were the staple fats used in most American homes. Somewhere around 1950, butter and lard dropped away from being the fats of choice in the western diet. At the same time more vegetable and seed oils as well as oleo (margarine) showed up on grocery shelves and were embraced as "healthy" alternatives.

These new vegetable and seed oils were all high in omega-6 fatty acids and much lower in Omega -3 fatty acids. We now know that omega-6 fatty acids can cause inflammation in the body when they are not consumed in a balanced ratio with Omega-3's. The current low fat diet recommendations encourage the use of vegetable and seed oils (polyunsaturated fats or PUFA's) with the end result being a typical western diet includes 15 to 20 times more than the recommended amount of Omega-6 fatty acids.[30]

Chronic inflammation slows down weight loss and suppresses autophagy. It can also cause stalls. No wonder so many well-intentioned dieters end up high and dry on a plateau feeling discouraged. Also, oils high in PUFA are not suitable for cooking. They oxidize at higher temperatures and become a further source of inflammation!

Then there's margarine. It is usually made using hydrogenated vegetable and seed oils and contains trans-fats which are produced when hydrogen molecules are added to liquid oils. Hydrogenation solidifies liquid oils and makes margarines spreadable. In general: the more solid a margarine, the higher its trans-fat content. Unfortunately, margarine has been viewed as the dieter's best choice for the better part of the past 60 years!

---

30 Totsch, Stacie K., Waite, Maegan E., Sorge, Robert E. *Dietary Influence on Pain via the Immune System, Chapter 15*. Progress in Molecular Biology and Translational Science, Volume 131. Pages, 435-569. Retrieved from https://www.sciencedirect.com/science/article/pii/S1877117314000283?via%3Dihub on 28/04/2018

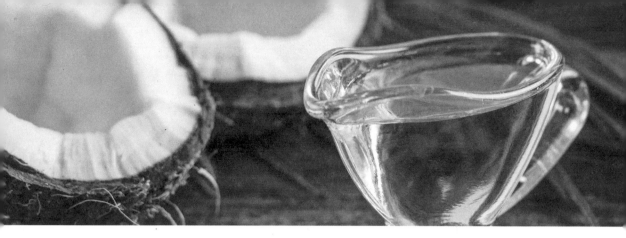

Pretty well everyone now agrees that trans-fats are just plain bad for you. Study after study has shown them to be a major culprit in causing heart disease and stroke because they raise your bad cholesterol (LDL) and lower the good cholesterol (HDL). Eating trans-fats also creates a higher risk for developing Type 2 diabetes.[31]

Add to this the fact that many food products include partially hydrogenated oils and you have a ticking trans-fat time bomb. Thankfully numerous scientific studies have finally convinced governments that action must be taken to protect the health of citizens.

In 2006, a Canadian Task Force on Trans-fat recommended that the health of Canadian people be protected with new formal regulations. This has led to a ban, making it illegal for manufacturers to include partially hydrogenated oils in all food products. The ban comes into effect in September, 2018.[32] Similarly in the US: "By June 18, 2018, human food must no longer contain partially hydrogenated oils for uses that have not been otherwise authorized by FDA."[33]

Look for and use fats that contain a high amount of saturated fatty acids, also called SFA's. Avoid those higher in polyunsaturated fat (PUFA) content whenever you can. The essential fatty-acids contained in PUFA's are important in a healthy diet but it's also important that these "essentials" be eaten in the correct proportions, one part omega-6 to 4 parts omega-3 (1:4). Most seed and vegetable oils are higher in Omega -6 and so we recommend avoiding them.

My recommended list of fats high in saturated fatty acids and lower in polyunsaturated fats (and their uses) follows:

- MCT oil (97% SFA, less than 1% PUFA) Can be heated - *use at low to moderate temperature, no higher than 320 F*

- Coconut oil (92% SFA, 1.9% PUFA) *Can be heated - use for cooking at higher temperatures*

- Cocoa butter (60% SFA, 3% PUFA) *Can be heated - use for cooking at higher temperatures*

- Duck Fat (25% SFA, 13% PUFA) *Can be heated -use for cooking at higher temperatures*

- Extra-virgin olive oil (14% SFA, 9.9% PUFA) *Use only at low heat temperatures or at room temperature as in salad dressings*

- Palm Kernel Oil (82% SFA, 2% PUFA) *Can be heated - use for cooking at higher temperatures*

---

31 *Article title: Trans Fat.* Retrieved from: https://healthyforgood.heart.org/eat-smart/articles/trans-fat retrieved on: 28/04/2018

32 Beck, Leslie. *What You Need To Know about Trans-fats and why they are being banned. Retrieved from: https://www.theglobeandmail.com/life/health-and-fitness/health/what-you-need-to-know-about-trans-fats-and-why-they-are-being-banned/article36317373/ Retrieved on: 28/04/2018*

33 *Final Determination Regarding Partially Hydrogenated Oils (Removing Trans-fats)*Retrieved from: https://www.fda.gov/Food/IngredientsPackagingLabeling/FoodAdditivesIngredients/ucm449162.htm Retrieved on 28/04/2014

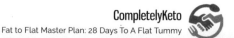

CompletelyKeto

Fat to Flat Master Plan: 28 Days To A Flat Tummy

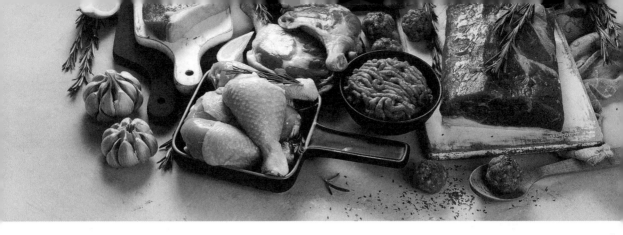

Meat

So, here's a bit more information about choosing organic, pastured meat. When I say "pastured" I mean meat from animals, like beef cattle and sheep (lamb) that have been allowed to graze on grass. This provides a natural diet for these animals. It's only in the last 60 years or so that American farmers have switched to feeding their livestock a predominantly corn based diet along with some other grains (it's cheaper). During this period we have seen rates of colon cancer soaring. Many believe this is due to over-consumption of red meat but it isn't so ...

In Argentina, where folks eat a twice as much red meat (beef), the rate of colon cancer is actually half of what we find in the US. So what's the difference? Well, Argentinean farmers are still pasturing their beef. When cattle are allowed to graze in a pasture the end result is meat that's better for you.

Grass-fed, raised-without-antibiotics meats are starting to appear on main-stream supermarket shelves in North America. As well, local farmers markets can be a good source of quality meats. Direct purchase from local organic farmers is also an option for many. There are also some internet based businesses that will actually deliver organic meats right to your door. Game meats are also a good source of healthy protein.

Red meat is limited to no more than 2 servings per week, and on the menu plan I've included it only once. Those of you who are eating left-overs on some days may eat red meat twice in a week.

- Bear
- Beef
- Bison (buffalo)
- Elk
- Goat
- Lamb
- Moose
- Rabbit
- Venison
- Eggs

I understand that some off you may be sensitive to eggs and will need to employ an egg replacer. The only egg replacer that can be used on the Fat to Flat Master Plan eating plan is made with grass-fed gelatin. Make a keto-friendly egg replacer by dissolving 1 T of grass-fed gelatin in 2 T of room temperature water. Add 2 T hot water and stir.

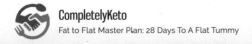

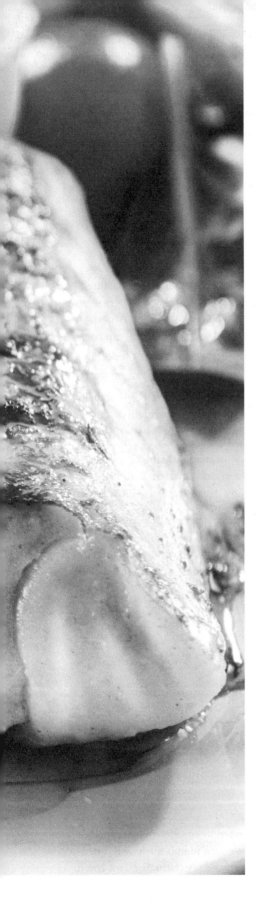

- Chicken eggs
- Duck eggs
- Goose eggs
- Ostrich eggs
- Quail eggs

High fat and/or fermented dairy products

Adding some dairy products (from grass fed cows) to your menu can add interest and flavor but I recommend keeping it to a minimum.

- Kefir
- Full fat yogurt

Small amount of hard, aged cheese, occasionally

Poultry

Choose free-range raised poultry with (no antibiotics) or game poultry.

- Chicken
- Duck
- Goose
- Game hen
- Ostrich
- Partridge
- Pheasant
- Quail
- Squab
- Turkey

Fish

- Ahi Ahi
- Catfish
- Cod
- Haddock
- Halibut
- Herring
- Hake

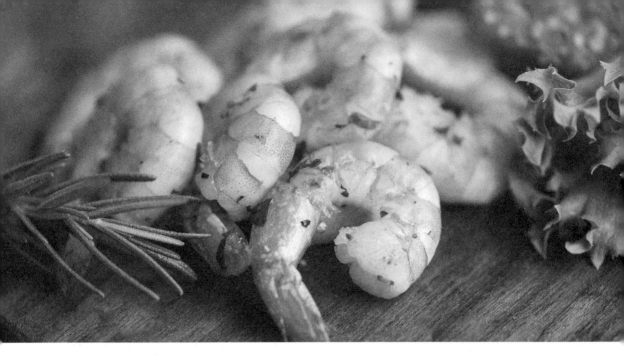

Fish (continued)

- Mackerel
- Mahi mahi
- Salmon
- Sardines
- Snapper
- Swordfish
- Tilapia
- Trout
- Tuna
- Walleye
- White fish

Seafood

- Clams
- Crab
- Lobster
- Mussels
- Oyster
- Prawn
- Scallop
- Scampi
- Shrimp

Fruit

In truth, the majority of fruit is very high in natural sugars so their carbohydrate count is too high for them to be included in a ketogenic eating plan.

However there are a few fruits we can include and mostly they are the ones we don't usually think of when considering fruit. Here's a list of the fruits you can include on Keto Express:

- Avocado
- Lemon
- Lime
- Eggplant
- Capers
- Olives
- Zucchini
- Tomato (keep this to a minimum)

Vegetables

- Arugula
- Asparagus
- Green or yellow beans
- Bok choy
- Broccoli

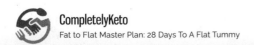

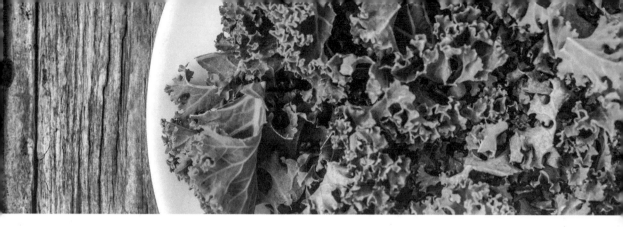

Vegetables (continued)

- Cabbage
- Cauliflower
- Celery
- Collard greens
- Endive
- Garlic
- Kale
- Kelp
- Lettuce
- Mushrooms
- Onions (scallions, red, yellow, white)
- Peppers
- Radishes
- Rutabaga
- Seaweed (Nori)
- Spinach
- Swiss chard
- Watercress

Vegetables to eat in smaller quantities

We've included the following vegetables but urge you to use them in smaller amounts as they are higher in carbohydrates than the veggies in the above list.

- Brussels sprouts
- Green beans
- Pumpkin

Beverages

Coffee drinking should be kept to a minimum; no more than 2 cups a day (this includes your 2 allowed Bullet Proof Coffees).

Caffeine can interfere with weight-loss for some people.

If you are in a stall try cutting out caffeine completely (this means coffee, black tea and green tea).

Make sure to drink plenty of water daily. If you can, drink reverse osmosis water.

- Kombucha
- Hunn Kombucha Tea
- Green tea with ginger
- Ginseng tea
- Oolong tea
- Tangerine Peel Tea
- Banyon Detox Tea
- A variety of other Green teas as desired
- Herbal tea
- Black tea
- Organic coffee
- Organic water processed decaffeinated coffee
- Mineral water
- Water
- Natural Sweeteners

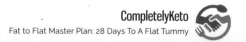

CompletelyKeto
Fat to Flat Master Plan: 28 Days To A Flat Tummy

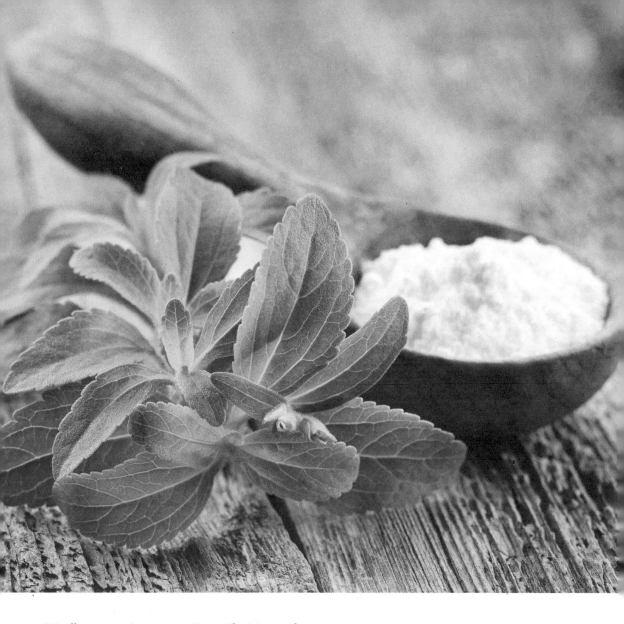

We allow two sweeteners on Fat to Flat Master Plan:

- Erythritol (natural sweetener found in some fermented foods and fruits)
- Liquid Stevia (use the liquid stevia not the granular because the granulated stevia contains maltodextrin which has an extremely high glycemic index)

Stevia Glycerate (has a thick honey-like texture and tends to not have a bitter after-taste like some other forms of stevia)

Powdered stevia (very concentrated powder – a little bit goes a long way!)

I use liquid (or powdered) stevia in most of the recipes that require some sweetening, however erythritol is allowed. It is a sugar alcohol that is found in some fruits and fermented foods. Commercially available Erythritol is made from corn. Look for a non-GMO Erythritol if you choose to use this sweetener. It's worth noting that not everyone tolerates erythritol well. It can cause diarrhea, headache and stomach ache in some people. So if you are new to using Erythritol use it sparingly until you see how you react.

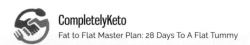

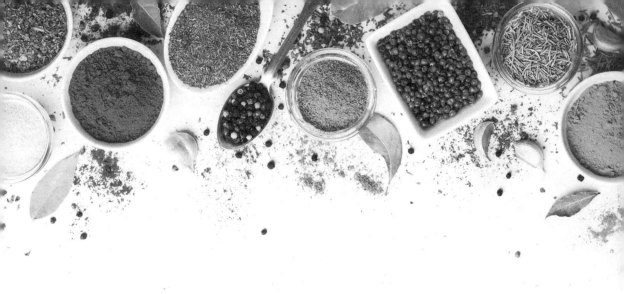

Herbs and Spices

Herbs and spices provide superb nutritional value and add flavor. Use them often!

- Anise
- Basil
- Bay leaf
- Black pepper
- Caraway
- Cardamom
- Cayenne pepper
- Celery seed
- Chervil
- Chili pepper
- Chives
- Cilantro
- Cinnamon
- Cloves
- Coriander
- Cumin
- Curry
- Dill
- Fenugreek

- Galangal
- Garlic
- Ginger
- Lemongrass
- Licorice
- Mace
- Marjoram
- Mint
- Mustard seeds
- Oregano
- Paprika
- Parsley
- Peppermint
- Rosemary
- Saffron
- Sage
- Spearmint
- Star anise
- Tarragon
- Thyme
- Turmeric
- Vanilla beans

 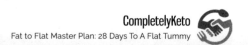

Flavor enhancers, sauces and other canned goods

Learn to read labels and then read them all the time. Choose products with no added sugars. It's possible to find things like basic tomato sauce and tomato paste that are made with simple keto-friendly ingredients but you have to be vigilant!

- Apple cider vinegar
- White vinegar
- Unseasoned rice vinegar *(no sugar added)*
- Gluten free tamari sauce
- Fish sauce *(no sugar added)*
- Boxed (organic) beef, chicken, turkey, fish and vegetable broths
- Canned anchovies
- Canned coconut milk *(full-fat)*
- Canned oysters
- Canned sardines
- Canned salmon
- Canned tuna
- Capers
- Fermented pickles *(no sugar added)*
- Fermented sauerkraut *(no sugar added)*
- Tomato sauce *(no sugar added)*
- Tomato paste *(no sugar added)*
- Hot sauce *(no sugar added)*
- Ketchup *(no sugar added)*
- Canned artichokes
- Olives

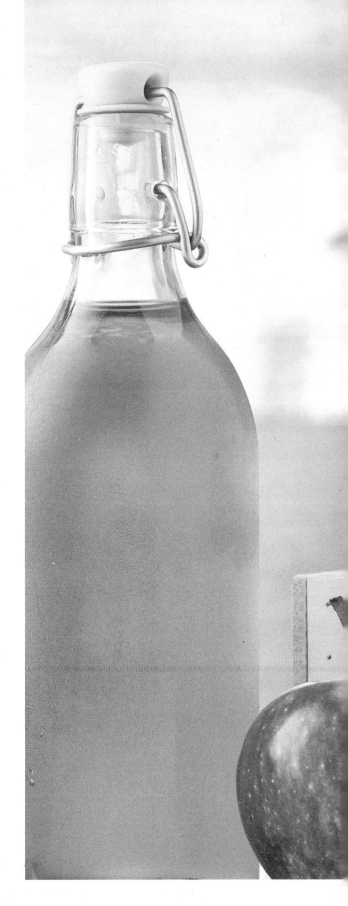

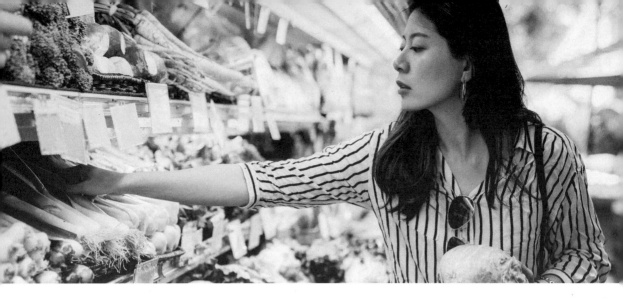

Chapter VI: Plan for Success

The Transition

You will need to take some easy actions before beginning this Fat to Flat Master Plan program to get yourself, your home and your work space ready for success. But success isn't happenstance; the transition into the keto lifestyle takes a bit of planning.

One obvious trick for success is to have your eating plan for each day already mapped out along with the needed ingredients handy and ready. This is why Fat to Flat Master Plan includes menu plans for each day, the recipes that go along with the menu plan and full lists for simplified grocery shopping because I know you need to plan for success. Read on for practical tips, helpful advice and easy actions you can take to get ready for success.

Preparing your pantry and kitchen ...

If you want to have success with your keto eating plan it's important to clear your kitchen of foods that are not allowed. Get rid of those half empty cereal and cracker boxes. Put away anything that may tempt you to stray from your new resolve. Place bags of sugar, flour and other baking supplies into a large tote with a tight fitting lid and store these things away from your daily kitchen routines; maybe even give them to a friend that likes to bake. Whatever you do, just don't keep these items where you can see them daily. Visuals are important.

"Out of sight, out of mind"

While bowls of nicely displayed fruit may be pleasing to the eye they could easily be your undoing. You know the old saying "out of sight, out of mind"? Well this adage definitely applies to what needs to happen on your kitchen counters and inside your cupboards and/or pantry. The same applies to the foods you are actually allowed to eat on Fat to Flat Master Plan. Leaving them out and visible can trigger mindless eating. Meals, beverages consumed and tea breaks should be planned. When it's time to eat, that meal deserves your full attention. It's far too easy to grab something and scarf it down simply because it's there, in front of you.

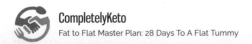

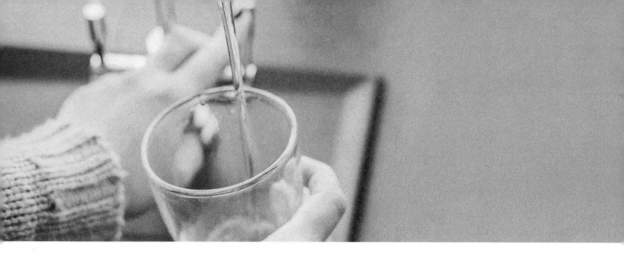

Make it easy to stay well hydrated

Drinking plenty of fluids is recommended and stocking up on a variety of organic teas and coffee, sugar free electrolyte drinks and organic chicken and beef bone broth is a must. Having a good supply of allowed beverages on hand makes hydration easy.

I also suggest keeping a small, juice-sized glass by the sink. Remember we already looked at how habits are formed in chapter one? Every time you find yourself in the kitchen it will be easy to establish the new habit of having a quick drink of water. Soon you will be doing it several times a day! Just seeing the glass waiting by the sink will eventually act as your cue to enjoy some sips of cool fresh water.

If you don't fancy the taste of water directly from the tap you can purchase one of the many filtered water pitchers that are available in stores. Keeping filtered water handy on the counter makes it easier to drink water regularly throughout the day.

Savor every mouthful!

A ketogenic diet requires some shifting in how you prepare meals and a willingness to try some new recipes. Meals can be both healthy and tasty. In fact, if you don't like what you are eating then stop and find something you do enjoy. While this doesn't happen often, when trying out a new recipe I've occasionally prepared a meal that just didn't measure up (at least according to my taste buds). Early on in my keto journey I decided that I would "savor every mouthful" and I've stuck to this decision faithfully.

This has meant that I've had to change some old programming about wasting food. As hard as it has been for me to scrape food from my plate into the organic recycling bin at my house, I've stuck with my resolve. If it doesn't taste good to me, I don't eat it; simple as that! Luckily I enjoy eggs, and since I always have them on hand in the fridge, when it's been necessary I've been able to whip up an omelet to replace a kitchen experiment that didn't quite work out.

Shopping for harder to find items

I know that some of you will have challenges finding some of the items I'm recommending like the Ayurvedic Tea powder for making the tea I want you to drink daily at bedtime or the bentonite clay for the poultice that I highly recommend. Everything that isn't found close by in your community can easily be found online and I've provided some links to make online shopping a bit easier. However, the reality of shopping online means you will have to plan ahead so these items, necessary for success, will arrive and be on hand when you are ready to start the program.

 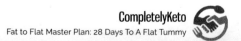

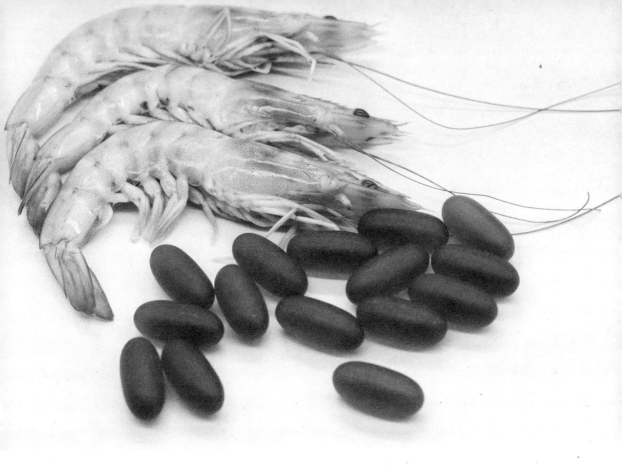

Here's a shopping list of supplements and other items to purchase from the local pharmacy (or online) ahead of time:

- Castor Oil (if doing the Castor Oil Cleanse on day #1)
- Triphala Powder (for Triphala Bedtime Drink)
- Human grade Bentonite Clay (optional)
- Home Cortisol Test Kit (optional)
- Electrolyte Powder Mix (if making your own electrolyte drinks)
- Magnesium Glycinate
- Vitamin D
- Full Spectrum Enzymes
- Probiotic (with Lactobaccillus and Bifidobacterium)
- Fish Oil
- Krill oil

The following items will assist in making your own fermented foods and are easily purchased from online sources or at the local hardware store:

- Fermenting Lids
- Glass Ferment Weight
- Wide Mouth Glass Mason Jars in a variety of sizes (pint, quart and/or gallon)

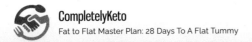

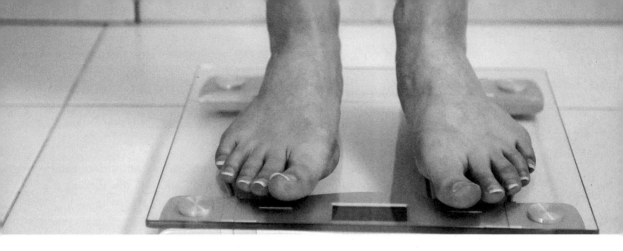

Chapter VII: The 28 Day Menu Plan

Do your homework first!

I know you are excited to get started but there are a few things I recommend before diving in. Read through all the chapters of this book so you understand the principles and science behind the ketogenic lifestyle. The Fat to Flat Master Plan plan combines ketogenic eating with a focus on gut health. Understanding the food choices in the menu plan that will help heal and maintain a healthy digestive tract will help you to stay committed throughout this month-long program.

Familiarize yourself with the concept of intermittent fasting and why it works so successfully with a ketogenic meal plan for those wanting to lose weight while gaining energy. Consult with your doctor if you have any medical concerns then make a firm decision to commit to one month of Fat to Flat Master Plan. Now print the calendar style, one-page menu plan and put it somewhere in the kitchen where it will be visible at a glance.

Two more things:

- Weigh yourself, record your weight then put your scales away for the month!
- Measure yourself around the chest, waist, hips, thighs (around both when standing with them together), around one thigh alone and around the upper arm

You will repeat this process at the end of the 4 week program and I feel sure you will be pleased with the results!

A word or two about substitutions ...

If what's listed on the menu plan doesn't appeal, swapping one meal for another is allowed; with one caveat. You must only substitute using recipes that are provided on the program. If you prefer one meal over another then that's what you should have. If the spice profile of a dish doesn't suit, then change it up for something that does appeal. The main thing here is to enjoy the meals you eat.

I expect some of you will be cooking for a family while others prepare food for just themselves. Most of the recipes provided will serve four adults. If you are making food for yourself you will either have to alter the recipe or freeze the extra portions for another day. You could also alter the menu plan by eating the leftovers next day. Changing the menu plan is always an option. I just want you to use it as a guide. And as already stated, only use the recipes provided if making changes!

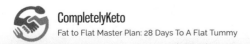

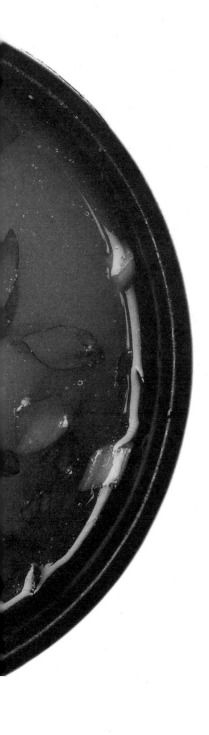

Week 1: Day #1 (Sunday)

The 28 day program starts with the Castor Oil Cleanse or OMAD, your choice.

If doing OMAD, start your day with Harlan's Anti-inflammatory Drink followed by a brisk 30-minute walk. Skip this if doing the Castor Oil Cleanse (must be done on an empty stomach).

Menu for the day:

- No breakfast or lunch
- Dinner: Light meal of Miso Soup and choice of steamed vegetables (from the allowed list) if you've chosen to do the cleanse. If you followed the OMAD protocol then you may have: Tofu and Bok Choy Stir-fry
- End your day with: Bedtime Triphala Drink

*drink 5 C of metabolic herbal tea/day: 8 a.m., 10 a.m., 2 p.m., 4 p.m. and 8 p.m.

**If doing OMAD you may drink these other allowed beverages to keep hydrated throughout the day: bullet proof coffee (no more than 2), kombucha, organic broth, black water-processed decaffeinated coffee, electrolyte drinks, water & herbal teas throughout the day.

*** If taking the Castor Oil Cleanse you may sip on kombucha, organic broth, black water-processed decaffeinated coffee, electrolyte drinks, water & herbal teas once evacuation of the bowels has ended.

Week 1: Day #2 (Monday)

Start your day with Harlan's Anti-inflammatory Drink followed by a brisk 30 minute walk.

Menu for the day:

- Breakfast: Eggs, Spinach and Smoked Salmon Breakfast Plate
- Lunch: Smoked Chicken (or Smoked Turkey) Sandwich with Fermented Dill Pickle
- Dinner: Turkey Keilbasa Oktoberfest Stew
- Finish your day with: Bedtime Triphala Drink

*drink 5 C of metabolic herbal tea/day: 8 a.m., 10 a.m., 2p.m., 4 p.m. and 8 p.m.

**Drink other allowed beverages to keep hydrated throughout the day: kombucha, organic broth, black Bullet Proof Coffee (only 2/day), black water-processed decaffeinated coffee, electrolyte drinks, water, tea, green teas & herbal teas.

CompletelyKeto
Fat to Flat Master Plan: 28 Days To A Flat Tummy

Week 1: Day #3 (Tuesday)

Start your day with Harlan's Anti- inflammatory Drink followed by a brisk 30 minute walk.

Menu for the day:

- Breakfast: <u>Strawberry Smoothie</u>
- Lunch: <u>Tuna, Avocado and Tomato Salad</u> with <u>Fermented Cauliflower</u>
- Dinner: <u>Citrus Thyme Roasted Chicken</u> and <u>Keto Tabouleh</u>
- Finish your day with: Bedtime Triphala Drink

drink 5 C of metabolic herbal tea/day: 8 a.m., 10 a.m., 2p.m., 4 p.m. and 8 p.m.

**Drink other allowed beverages to keep hydrated throughout the day: kombucha, organic broth, black Bullet Proof Coffee (only 2/day), black water-processed decaffeinated coffee, electrolyte drinks, water, tea, green teas & herbal teas.*

Week 1: Day #4 (Wednesday)

Start your day with Harlan's Anti-inflammatory Drink followed by a brisk 30 minute walk.

Menu for the day:

- Breakfast: <u>Fried Egg, Arugula and Asparagus Breakfast Plate</u>
- Lunch: <u>Chicken Lunch Salad</u> with 1 or 2 <u>Fermented Peppers</u>
- Dinner: <u>Teriyaki Salmon Fillet</u> with Kimchi Fried "Rice"
- Finish your day with: Bedtime Triphala Drink

drink 5 C of metabolic herbal tea/day: 8 a.m., 10 a.m., 2p.m., 4 p.m. and 8 p.m.

**Drink other allowed beverages to keep hydrated throughout the day: kombucha, organic broth, black Bullet Proof Coffee (only 2/day), black water-processed decaffeinated coffee, electrolyte drinks, water, tea, green teas & herbal teas.*

Week 1: Day #5 (Thursday)

Start your day with Harlan's Anti-inflammatory Drink followed by a brisk 30 minute walk.

Menu for the day:

- Breakfast: <u>Blueberry Smoothie</u>
- Lunch: <u>Basic Green Salad</u> and <u>Deviled Dilly Eggs</u> with a <u>Fermented Sour Dill Pickle</u>
- Dinner: <u>Easy Shrimp/Artichoke Tacos</u> garnished with <u>Fermented Salsa Verde</u> (if desired)
- Finish your day with: Bedtime Triphala Drink

drink 5 C of metabolic herbal tea/day: 8 a.m., 10 a.m., 2p.m., 4 p.m. and 8 p.m.

**Drink other allowed beverages to keep hydrated throughout the day: kombucha, organic broth, black Bullet Proof Coffee (only 2/day), black water-processed decaffeinated coffee, electrolyte drinks, water, tea, green teas & herbal teas.*

Week 1: Day #6 (Friday)

Start your day with Harlan's Anti-inflammatory Drink followed by a brisk 30 minute walk.

Menu for the day:

- Breakfast: <u>Sauerkraut, Cabbage and Turkey Bacon Stir-fry</u>
- Lunch: <u>Hot and Sour Soup</u>
- Dinner: <u>Tex Mex Tempeh and Zucchini</u> with <u>Fermented Red Salsa</u> on the side
- Finish your day with: Bedtime Triphala Drink

drink 5 C of metabolic herbal tea/day: 8 a.m., 10 a.m., 2p.m., 4 p.m. and 8 p.m.

**Drink other allowed beverages to keep hydrated throughout the day: black Bullet Proof Coffee (only 2/day), black water-processed decaffeinated coffee, electrolyte drinks, water, tea, green teas & herbal teas.*

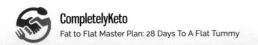

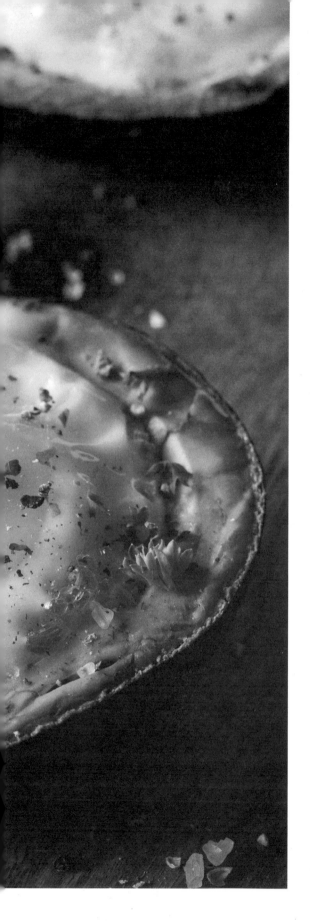

Week 1: Day #7 (Saturday)

Start your day with Harlan's Anti-inflammatory Drink followed by a brisk 30 minute walk.

Menu for the day:

- Breakfast: Kimchi Fried "Rice" and Egg Breakfast Bowl
- Lunch: Tom Kha (coconut/ salmon soup)
- Dinner: Keto-style Beef Bourguignon on Cauliflower Mash and Stir-fried Shredded Cabbage
- Finish your day with: Bedtime Triphala Drink

drink 5 C of metabolic herbal tea/day: 8 a.m., 10 a.m., 2p.m., 4 p.m. and 8 p.m.

**Drink other allowed beverages to keep hydrated throughout the day: kombucha, organic broth, black Bullet Proof Coffee (only 2/day), black water-processed decaffeinated coffee, electrolyte drinks, water, tea, green teas & herbal teas.*

Week 2: Day #8 (Sunday)

Start your day with Harlan's Anti-inflammatory Drink followed by a brisk 30 minute walk.

Menu for the day:

- Breakfast: Herbed Baked Egg in Avocado
- Lunch: Smoked Salmon Salad with Fermented Sour Dill Pickles
- Dinner: Coconut Cauliflower Chicken Curry with Homemade Fermented Hot Sauce on the side
- Finish your day with: Bedtime Triphala Drink

drink 5 C of metabolic herbal tea/day: 8 a.m., 10 a.m., 2p.m., 4 p.m. and 8 p.m.

**Drink other allowed beverages to keep hydrated throughout the day: kombucha, organic broth, black Bullet Proof Coffee (only 2/day), black water-processed decaffeinated coffee, electrolyte drinks, water, tea, green teas & herbal teas.*

CompletelyKeto

Fat to Flat Master Plan: 28 Days To A Flat Tummy

Week 2: Day #9 (Monday)

Today is an OMAD day

Start your day with Harlan's Anti-inflammatory Drink followed by a brisk 30 minute walk.

Menu for the day:

- No breakfast or lunch
- Dinner: Braised Haddock with Fried Cauliflower "Rice" and a few fermented pickles of choice
- Finish your day with: Bedtime Triphala Drink

drink 5 C of metabolic herbal tea/day: 8 a.m., 10 a.m., 2p.m., 4 p.m. and 8 p.m.

**Drink other allowed beverages to keep hydrated throughout the day: kombucha, black Bullet Proof Coffee (only 2/day), black water-processed decaffeinated coffee, electrolyte drinks, water, tea, green teas & herbal teas.*

Week 2: Day #10 (Tuesday)

Start your day with Harlan's Anti-inflammatory Drink followed by a brisk 30 minute walk.

Menu for the day:

- Breakfast: Cucumber Kefir
- Lunch: Miso Soup and Smoked Turkey Sandwich
- Dinner: Easy Rustic Chicken Roast with Roasted Brussels Sprouts and Fermented Cauliflower
- Finish your day with: Bedtime Triphala Drink

drink 5 C of metabolic herbal tea/day: 8 a.m., 10 a.m., 2p.m., 4 p.m. and 8 p.m.

**Drink other allowed beverages to keep hydrated throughout the day: kombucha, organic broth, black Bullet Proof Coffee (only 2/day), black water-processed decaffeinated coffee, electrolyte drinks, water, tea, green teas & herbal teas.*

Week 2: Day #11 (Wednesday)

Start your day with Harlan's Anti-inflammatory Drink followed by a brisk 30 minute walk.

Menu for the day:

- Breakfast: Perfectly Poached Eggs on Stir-fried Shredded Cabbage
- Lunch: Sauerkraut Chicken Soup
- Dinner: Tex Mex Tempeh and Zucchini with Fermented Red Salsa on the side
- Finish your day with: Bedtime Triphala Drink

drink 5 C of metabolic herbal tea/day: 8 a.m., 10 a.m., 2p.m., 4 p.m. and 8 p.m.

**Drink other allowed beverages to keep hydrated throughout the day: black Bullet Proof Coffee (only 2/day), black water-processed decaffeinated coffee, electrolyte drinks, water, tea, green teas & herbal teas.*

Week 2: Day #12 (Thursday)

Start your day with Harlan's Anti-inflammatory Drink followed by a brisk 30 minute walk.

Menu for the day:

- Breakfast: Instant Pot Greek Yogurt with ½ C fresh sliced strawberries
- Lunch: Chicken Lunch Salad with 1 or 2 Fermented Peppers
- Dinner: Baked Hake with Rosemary and Lemon and Garlic Zucchini Noodles
- Finish your day with: Bedtime Triphala Drink

drink 5 C of metabolic herbal tea/day: 8 a.m., 10 a.m., 2p.m., 4 p.m. and 8 p.m.

**Drink other allowed beverages to keep hydrated throughout the day: kombucha, organic broth, black Bullet Proof Coffee (only 2/day), black water-processed decaffeinated coffee, electrolyte drinks, water, tea, green teas & herbal teas.*

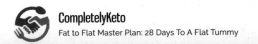

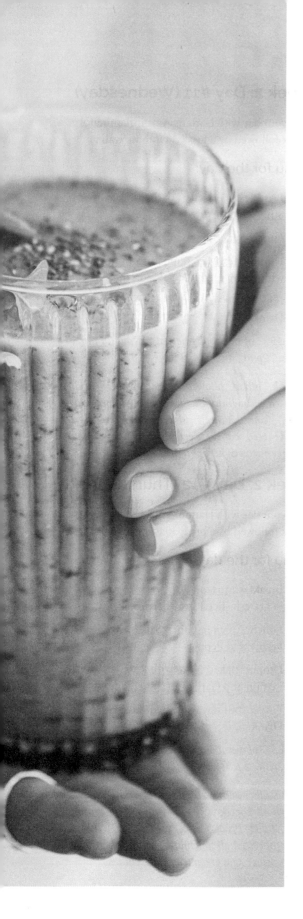

Week 2: Day #13 (Friday)

Start your day with Harlan's Anti-inflammatory Drink followed by a brisk 30 minute walk.

Menu for the day:

- Breakfast: <u>Scrambled Eggs with Mushroom Compote</u>
- Lunch: <u>Egg Salad Sandwich</u> with fermented pickles of choice
- Dinner: <u>Lamb Stew</u> with <u>Cauliflower Mash</u>
- Finish your day with: Bedtime Triphala Drink

drink 5 C of metabolic herbal tea/day: 8 a.m., 10 a.m., 2p.m., 4 p.m. and 8 p.m.

**Drink other allowed beverages to keep hydrated throughout the day: kombucha, organic broth, black Bullet Proof Coffee (only 2/day), black water-processed decaffeinated coffee, electrolyte drinks, water, tea, green teas & herbal teas.*

Week 2: Day #14 (Saturday)

Start your day with Harlan's Anti-inflammatory Drink followed by a brisk 30 minute walk.

Menu for the day:

- Breakfast: <u>Green Morning Smoothie</u>
- Lunch: <u>Tuna, Avocado and Tomato Salad</u> with <u>Fermented Peppers</u> on the side
- Dinner: <u>Chicken Thighs and Baby Bok Choy</u> with Kimchi Fried "Rice" or <u>Daikon Kimchi-style Fermented Pickles</u>
- Finish your day with: Bedtime Triphala Drink

drink 5 C of metabolic herbal tea/day: 8 a.m., 10 a.m., 2p.m., 4 p.m. and 8 p.m.

**Drink other allowed beverages to keep hydrated throughout the day: kombucha, organic broth, black Bullet Proof Coffee (only 2/day), black water-processed decaffeinated coffee, electrolyte drinks, water, tea, green teas & herbal teas.*

Week 3: Day # 15 (Sunday)

Start your day with Harlan's Anti-inflammatory Drink followed by a brisk 30 minute walk.

Menu for the day:

- Breakfast: Tex Mex Baked Eggs
- Lunch: Tom Kha (coconut/ salmon soup)
- Dinner: Mushroom Tempeh Burger and Simple Roasted Veggie Salad
- Finish your day with: Bedtime Triphala Drink

drink 5 C of metabolic herbal tea/day: 8 a.m., 10 a.m., 2p.m., 4 p.m. and 8 p.m.

**Drink other allowed beverages to keep hydrated throughout the day: kombucha, organic broth, black Bullet Proof Coffee (only 2/day), black water-processed decaffeinated coffee, electrolyte drinks, water, tea, green teas & herbal teas.*

Week 3: Day # 16 (Monday)

Today is an OMAD day

Start your day with Harlan's Anti-inflammatory Drink followed by a brisk 30 minute walk.

Menu for the day:

- No breakfast or lunch
- Dinner: Simple Keto Hunan Chicken with Cauliflower "Rice" or Kimchi Fried "Rice"
- Finish your day with: Bedtime Triphala Drink

drink 5 C of metabolic herbal tea/day: 8 a.m., 10 a.m., 2p.m., 4 p.m. and 8 p.m.

**Drink other allowed beverages to keep hydrated throughout the day: kombucha, organic broth, black Bullet Proof Coffee (only 2/day), black water-processed decaffeinated coffee, electrolyte drinks, water, tea, green teas & herbal teas.*

Week 3: Day #17 (Tuesday)

Start your day with Harlan's Anti-inflammatory Drink followed by a brisk 30 minute walk.

Menu for the day:

- Breakfast: Glass of Homemade Kefir and ½ C sliced fresh strawberries
- Lunch: Smoked Turkey Sandwich and fermented pickle of choice
- Dinner: Citrus Thyme Roasted Chicken with Broccoli Salad
- Finish your day with: Bedtime Triphala Drink

drink 5 C of metabolic herbal tea/day: 8 a.m., 10 a.m., 2p.m., 4 p.m. and 8 p.m.

**Drink other allowed beverages to keep hydrated throughout the day: kombucha, organic broth, black Bullet Proof Coffee (only 2/day), black water-processed decaffeinated coffee, electrolyte drinks, water, tea, green teas & herbal teas.*

Week 3: Day #18 (Wednesday)

Start your day with Harlan's Anti-inflammatory Drink followed by a brisk 30 minute walk.

Menu for the day:

- Breakfast: Fried Egg, Arugula and Asparagus
- Lunch: Chicken Lunch Salad
- Dinner: Perfect Steak garnished with Fermented Salsa Verde on the side and Roasted Brussels Sprouts
- Finish your day with: Bedtime Triphala Drink

drink 5 C of metabolic herbal tea/day: 8 a.m., 10 a.m., 2p.m., 4 p.m. and 8 p.m.

**Drink other allowed beverages to keep hydrated throughout the day: kombucha, organic broth, black Bullet Proof Coffee (only 2/day), black water-processed decaffeinated coffee, electrolyte drinks, water, tea, green teas & herbal teas.*

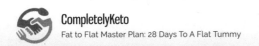

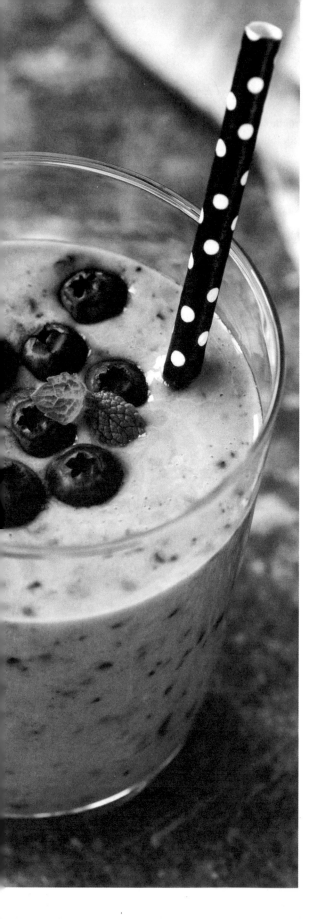

Week 3: Day #19 (Thursday)

Start your day with Harlan's Anti-inflammatory Drink followed by a brisk 30 minute walk.

Menu for the day:

- Breakfast: Blueberry Smoothie
- Lunch: Smoked Chicken Sandwich and Fermented Sour Dill Pickle
- Dinner: Sauerkraut, Cabbage and Turkey Bacon Stir-fry
- Finish your day with: Bedtime Triphala Drink

drink 5 C of metabolic herbal tea/day: 8 a.m., 10 a.m., 2p.m., 4 p.m. and 8 p.m.

**Drink other allowed beverages to keep hydrated throughout the day: kombucha, organic broth, black Bullet Proof Coffee (only 2/day), black water-processed decaffeinated coffee, electrolyte drinks, water, tea, green teas & herbal teas.*

Week 3: Day #20 (Friday)

Start your day with Harlan's Anti-inflammatory Drink followed by a brisk 30 minute walk.

Menu for the day:

- Breakfast: Eggs, Spinach and Smoked Salmon Breakfast Plate
- Lunch: Easy Shrimp/Artichoke Tacos with Fermented Red Salsa
- Dinner: Beef Sausage and Sauerkraut Skillet Dinner with Buffalo Cauliflower
- Finish your day with: Bedtime Triphala Drink

drink 5 C of metabolic herbal tea/day: 8 a.m., 10 a.m., 2p.m., 4 p.m. and 8 p.m.

**Drink other allowed beverages to keep hydrated throughout the day: kombucha, organic broth, black Bullet Proof Coffee (only 2/day), black water-processed decaffeinated coffee, electrolyte drinks, water, tea, green teas & herbal teas.*

Week 3: Day #21 (Saturday)

Start your day with Harlan's Anti-inflammatory Drink followed by a brisk 30 minute walk.

Menu for the day:

- Breakfast: Green Morning Smoothie
- Lunch: Sauerkraut Chicken Soup
- Dinner: Braised Haddock and Cauliflower "Rice"
- Finish your day with: Bedtime Triphala Drink

drink 5 C of metabolic herbal tea/day: 8 a.m., 10 a.m., 2p.m., 4 p.m. and 8 p.m.

**Drink other allowed beverages to keep hydrated throughout the day: kombucha, organic broth, black Bullet Proof Coffee (only 2/day), black water-processed decaffeinated coffee, electrolyte drinks, water, tea, green teas & herbal teas.*

Week 4: Day #22 (Sunday)

Start your day with Harlan's Anti-inflammatory Drink followed by a brisk 30 minute walk.

Menu for the day:

- Breakfast: Kimchi Fried "Rice" and Egg Breakfast Bowl
- Lunch: Miso Soup and Egg Salad Sandwich
- Dinner: Broccoli, Salmon Frittata and Basic Green Salad with fermented pickles of choice
- Finish your day with: Bedtime Triphala Drink

drink 5 C of metabolic herbal tea/day: 8 a.m., 10 a.m., 2p.m., 4 p.m. and 8 p.m.

**Drink other allowed beverages to keep hydrated throughout the day: kombucha, organic broth, black Bullet Proof Coffee (only 2/day), black water-processed decaffeinated coffee, electrolyte drinks, water, tea, green teas & herbal teas.*

Week 4: Day #23 (Monday)

Today is an OMAD day

Start your day with Harlan's Anti-inflammatory Drink followed by a brisk 30 minute walk.

Menu for the day:

- No breakfast or lunch
- Dinner: Green Bean/Tempeh Wok Dish with Fried Cauliflower "Rice"
- Finish your day with: Bedtime Triphala Drink

drink 5 C of metabolic herbal tea/day: 8 a.m., 10 a.m., 2p.m., 4 p.m. and 8 p.m.

**Drink other allowed beverages to keep hydrated throughout the day: kombucha, organic broth, black Bullet Proof Coffee (only 2/day), black water-processed decaffeinated coffee, electrolyte drinks, water, tea, green teas & herbal teas.*

Week 4: Day #24 (Tuesday)

Start your day with Harlan's Anti-inflammatory Drink followed by a brisk 30 minute walk.

Menu for the day:

- Breakfast: Cucumber Kefir
- Lunch: Basic Green Salad and Deviled Dilly Eggs with a Fermented Sour Dill Pickle
- Dinner: Turkey Keilbasa Oktoberfest Stew
- Finish your day with: Bedtime Triphala Drink

drink 5 C of metabolic herbal tea/day: 8 a.m., 10 a.m., 2p.m., 4 p.m. and 8 p.m.

**Drink other allowed beverages to keep hydrated throughout the day: kombucha, organic broth, black Bullet Proof Coffee (only 2/day), black water-processed decaffeinated coffee, electrolyte drinks, water, tea, green teas & herbal teas.*

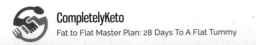

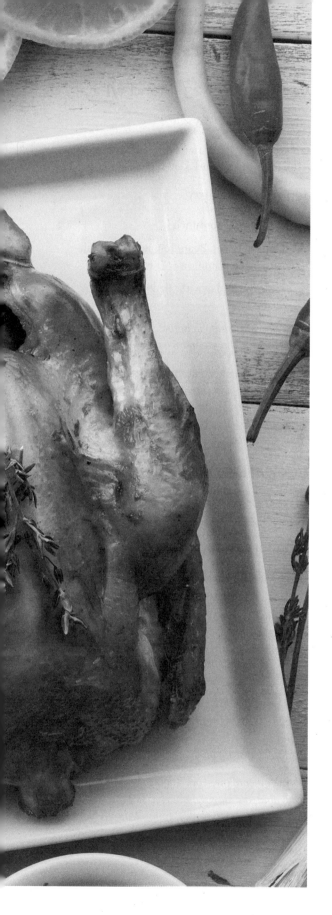

Week 4: Day #25 (Wednesday)

Start your day with Harlan's Anti-inflammatory Drink followed by a brisk 30 minute walk.

Menu for the day:

- Breakfast: Strawberry Smoothie
- Lunch: Tuna, Avocado and Tomato Salad with Fermented Cauliflower
- Dinner: Citrus Thyme Roasted Chicken and Keto Tabouleh
- Finish your day with: Bedtime Triphala Drink

drink 5 C of metabolic herbal tea/day: 8 a.m., 10 a.m., 2p.m., 4 p.m. and 8 p.m.

**Drink other allowed beverages to keep hydrated throughout the day: kombucha, organic broth, black Bullet Proof Coffee (only 2/day), black water-processed decaffeinated coffee, electrolyte drinks, water, tea, green teas & herbal teas.*

Week 4: Day #26 (Thursday)

Start your day with Harlan's Anti-inflammatory Drink followed by a brisk 30 minute walk.

Menu for the day:

- Breakfast: Sauerkraut, Cabbage and Turkey Bacon Stir-fry
- Lunch: Hot and Sour Soup
- Dinner: Tex Mex Tempeh and Zucchini with Fermented Red Salsa on the side
- Finish your day with: Bedtime Triphala Drink

drink 5 C of metabolic herbal tea/day: 8 a.m., 10 a.m., 2p.m., 4 p.m. and 8 p.m.

**Drink other allowed beverages to keep hydrated throughout the day: kombucha, organic broth, black Bullet Proof Coffee (only 2/day), black water-processed decaffeinated coffee, electrolyte drinks, water, tea, green teas & herbal teas.*

CompletelyKeto
Fat to Flat Master Plan: 28 Days To A Flat Tummy

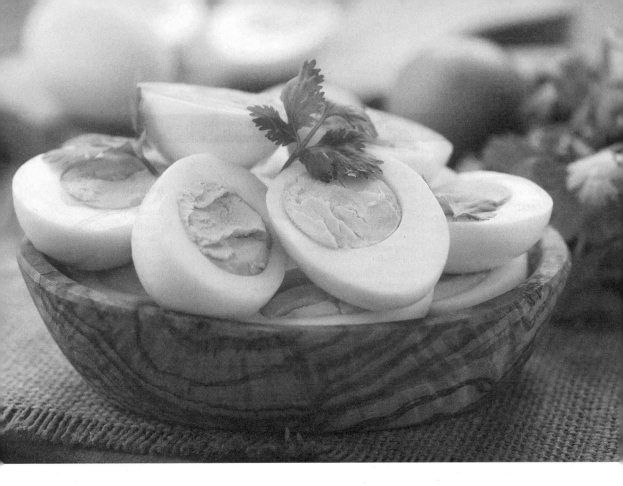

Week 4: Day #27 (Friday)

Start your day with Harlan's Anti-inflammatory Drink followed by a brisk 30 minute walk.

Menu for the day:

- Breakfast: Perfectly Boiled Eggs
- Lunch: Tom Kha (coconut/ salmon soup) and fermented pickles of choice
- Dinner: Keto-style Beef Bourguignon on Cauliflower Mash and Stir-fried Shredded Cabbage

drink 5 C of metabolic herbal tea/day: 8 a.m., 10 a.m., 2p.m., 4 p.m. and 8 p.m.

**Drink other allowed beverages to keep hydrated throughout the day: kombucha, organic broth, black Bullet Proof Coffee (only 2/day), black water-processed decaffeinated coffee, electrolyte drinks, water, tea, green teas & herbal teas.*

Week 4: Day #28 (Saturday)

Start your day with Harlan's Anti-inflammatory Drink followed by a brisk 30 minute walk.

Menu for the day:

- Breakfast: Blueberry Smoothie
- Lunch: Smoked Salmon Salad with Fermented Sour Dill Pickles
- Dinner: Chicken Thighs and Baby Bok Choy with Kimchi Fried "Rice" or Daikon Kimchi-style Fermented Pickles
- Finish your day with: Bedtime Triphala Drink

drink 5 C of metabolic herbal tea/day: 8 a.m., 10 a.m., 2p.m., 4 p.m. and 8 p.m.

**Drink other allowed beverages to keep hydrated throughout the day: kombucha, organic broth, black Bullet Proof Coffee (only 2/day), black water-processed decaffeinated coffee, electrolyte drinks, water, tea, green teas & herbal teas.*

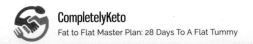

Meal Calendar:

Sunday	Monday	Tuesday	Wednesday
Day 1 Weigh yourself Measure yourself Put the scales away! **OMAD or Castor Oil Cleanse Dinner for OMAD:** Tofu and Bok Choy Stir-Fry **Dinner for Cleanse:** Miso Soup and Steamed Cauliflower and Broccoli **Bedtime:** Triphala Drink	**Day 2** Anti-inflammatory Drink and brisk 30 minute walk. **Breakfast:** Eggs, Spinach and Smoked Salmon Breakfast Plate **Lunch:** Smoked Chicken (or Smoked Turkey) Sandwich with Fermented Dill Pickle **Dinner:** Turkey Keilbasa Oktoberfest Stew **Bedtime:** Triphala Drink	**Day 3** Anti-inflammatory Drink and brisk 30 minute walk. **Breakfast:** Strawberry Smoothie **Lunch:** Tuna, Avocado and Tomato Salad with Fermented Cauliflower **Dinner:** Citrus Thyme Roasted Chicken and Keto Tabouleh **Bedtime:** Triphala Drink	**Day 4** Anti-inflammatory Drink and brisk 30 minute walk. **Breakfast:** Fried Egg, Arugula and Asparagus Breakfast Plate **Lunch:** Chicken Lunch Salad with 1 or 2 Fermented Peppers **Dinner:** Teriyaki Salmon Filet with Kimchi Fried "Rice" **Bedtime:** Triphala Drink
Day 8 Anti-inflammatory Drink and brisk 30 minute walk. **Breakfast:** Herbed Baked Egg in Avocado **Lunch:** Smoked Salmon Salad with Fermented Sour Dill Pickles **Dinner:** Coconut Cauliflower Chicken Curry with Homemade Fermented Hot Sauce on the side **Bedtime:** Triphala Drink	**Day 9** OMAD Anti-inflammatory Drink and brisk 30 minute walk. No breakfast and lunch **Dinner:** Braised Haddock with Fried Cauliflower "Rice" and a few fermented pickles of choice **Bedtime:** Triphala Drink	**Day 10** Anti-inflammatory Drink and brisk 30 minute walk. **Breakfast:** Cucumber Kefir **Lunch:** Miso Soup and Smoked Turkey Sandwich **Dinner:** Easy Rustic Chicken Roast with Roasted Brussel Sprouts and Fermented Cauliflower **Bedtime:** Triphala Drink	**Day 11** Anti-inflammatory Drink and brisk 30 minute walk. **Breakfast:** Perfectly Poached Eggs on Stir-fried Shredded Cabbage **Lunch:** Sauerkraut Chicken Soup **Dinner:** Tex Mex Tempeh and Zucchini with Fermented Red Salsa on the side **Bedtime:** Triphala Drink
Day 15 Anti-inflammatory Drink and brisk 30 minute walk. **Breakfast:** Tex Mex Baked Eggs **Lunch:** Tom Kha (coconut/salmon soup) **Dinner:** Mushroom Tempeh Burger and Simple Roasted Veggie Salad **Bedtime:** Triphala Drink	**Day 16** OMAD Anti-inflammatory Drink and brisk 30 minute walk. No breakfast and lunch **Dinner:** Simple Keto Hunan Chicken with Cauliflower "Rice" or Kimchi Fried "Rice" **Bedtime:** Triphala Drink	**Day 17** Anti-inflammatory Drink and brisk 30 minute walk. **Breakfast:** Homemade Kefir and ½ C sliced fresh strawberries **Lunch:** Smoked Turkey Sandwich and fermented pickle of choice **Dinner:** Citrus Thyme Roasted Chicken with Broccoli Salad **Bedtime:** Triphala Drink	**Day 18** Anti-inflammatory Drink and brisk 30 minute walk. **Breakfast:** Fried Egg, Arugula and Asparagus **Lunch:** Chicken Lunch Salad **Dinner:** Perfect Steak garnished with Fermented Salsa Verde on the side and Roasted Brussel Sprouts **Bedtime:** Triphala Drink
Day 22 Anti-inflammatory Drink and brisk 30 minute walk. **Breakfast:** Kimchi Fried "Rice" and Egg Breakfast Bowl **Lunch:** Miso Soup and Egg Salad Sandwich **Dinner:** Broccoli, Salmon Frittata and Basic Green Salad with fermented pickles of choice **Bedtime:** Triphala Drink	**Day 23** OMAD Anti-inflammatory Drink and brisk 30 minute walk. No breakfast and lunch **Dinner:** Green Bean/Tempeh Wok Dish with Fried Cauliflower "Rice" **Bedtime:** Triphala Drink	**Day 24** Anti-inflammatory Drink and brisk 30 minute walk. **Breakfast:** Cucumber Kefir **Lunch:** Basic Green Salad and Deviled Dilly Eggs with a Fermented Sour Dill Pickle **Dinner:** Turkey Keilbasa Oktoberfest Stew **Bedtime:** Triphala Drink	**Day 25** Anti-inflammatory Drink and brisk 30 minute walk. **Breakfast:** Strawberry Smoothie **Lunch:** Tuna, Avocado and Tomato Salad with Fermented Cauliflower **Dinner:** Citrus Thyme Roasted Chicken and Keto Tabouleh **Bedtime:** Triphala Drink

CompletelyKeto

Fat to Flat Master Plan: 28 Days To A Flat Tummy

Meal Calendar (continued):

Thursay	Friday	Saturday
Day 5 Anti-inflammatory Drink and brisk 30 minute walk. **Breakfast:** Blueberry Smoothie **Lunch:** Basic Green Salad and Deviled Dilly Eggs with a Fermented Sour Dill Pickle **Dinner:** Easy Shrimp/Artichoke Tacos garnished with Fermented Salsa Verde (if desired) **Bedtime:** Triphala Drink	**Day 6** Anti-inflammatory Drink and brisk 30 minute walk. **Breakfast:** Sauerkraut, Cabbage and Turkey Bacon Stir-fry **Lunch:** Hot and Sour Soup **Dinner:** Tex Mex Tempeh and Zucchini with Fermented Red Salsa on the side **Bedtime:** Triphala Drink	**Day 7** Anti-inflammatory Drink and brisk 30 minute walk. **Breakfast:** Kimchi Fried "Rice" and Egg Breakfast Bowl **Lunch:** Tom Kha (coconut/ salmon soup) **Dinner:** Keto-style Beef Bourguignon on Cauliflower Mash and Stir-fried Shredded Cabbage **Bedtime:** Triphala Drink
Day 12 Anti-inflammatory Drink and brisk 30 minute walk. **Breakfast:** Instant Pot Greek Yogurt with ½ C fresh sliced strawberries **Lunch:** Chicken Lunch Salad with 1 or 2 Fermented Peppers **Dinner:** Baked Hake with Rosemary and Lemon and Garlic Zucchini Noodles **Bedtime:** Triphala Drink	**Day 13** Anti-inflammatory Drink and brisk 30 minute walk. **Breakfast:** Scrambled Eggs with Mushroom Compote **Lunch:** Egg Salad Sandwich with fermented pickles of choice **Dinner:** Lamb Stew with Cauliflower Mash **Bedtime:** Triphala Drink	**Day 14** Anti-inflammatory Drink and brisk 30 minute walk. **Breakfast:** Green Morning Smoothie **Lunch:** Tuna, Avocado and Tomato Salad with Fermented Peppers on the side **Dinner:** Chicken Thighs and Baby Bok Choy with Kimchi Fried "Rice" or Daikon Kimchi-style Fermented Pickles **Bedtime:** Triphala Drink
Day 19 Anti-inflammatory Drink and brisk 30 minute walk. **Breakfast:** Blueberry Smoothie **Lunch:** Smoked Chicken Sandwich and Fermented Sour Dill Pickle **Dinner:** Sauerkraut, Cabbage and Turkey Bacon Stir-fry **Bedtime:** Triphala Drink	**Day 20** Anti-inflammatory Drink and brisk 30 minute walk. **Breakfast:** Eggs, Spinach and Smoked Salmon Breakfast Plate **Lunch:** Easy Shrimp/Artichoke Tacos with Fermented Red Salsa **Dinner:** Beef Sausage and Sauerkraut Skillet Dinner with Buffalo Cauliflower **Bedtime:** Triphala Drink	**Day 21** Anti-inflammatory Drink and brisk 30 minute walk. **Breakfast:** Green Morning Smoothie **Lunch:** Sauerkraut Chicken Soup **Dinner:** Braised Haddock and Cauliflower "Rice" **Bedtime:** Triphala Drink
Day 26 Anti-inflammatory Drink and brisk 30 minute walk. **Breakfast:** Sauerkraut, Cabbage and Turkey Bacon Stir-fry **Lunch:** Hot and Sour Soup **Dinner:** Tex Mex Tempeh and Zucchini with Fermented Red Salsa on the side **Bedtime:** Triphala Drink	**Day 27** Anti-inflammatory Drink and brisk 30 minute walk. **Breakfast:** Perfectly Boiled Eggs **Lunch:** Tom Kha (coconut/ salmon soup) and fermented pickles of choice **Dinner:** Keto-style Beef Bourguignon on Cauliflower Mash and Stir-fried Shredded Cabbage **Bedtime:** Triphala Drink	**Day 28** Anti-inflammatory Drink and brisk 30 minute walk. **Breakfast:** Blueberry Smoothie **Lunch:** Smoked Salmon Salad with Fermented Sour Dill Pickles **Dinner:** Chicken Thighs and Baby Bok Choy with Kimchi Fried "Rice" or Daikon Kimchi-style Fermented Pickles **Bedtime:** Triphala Drink

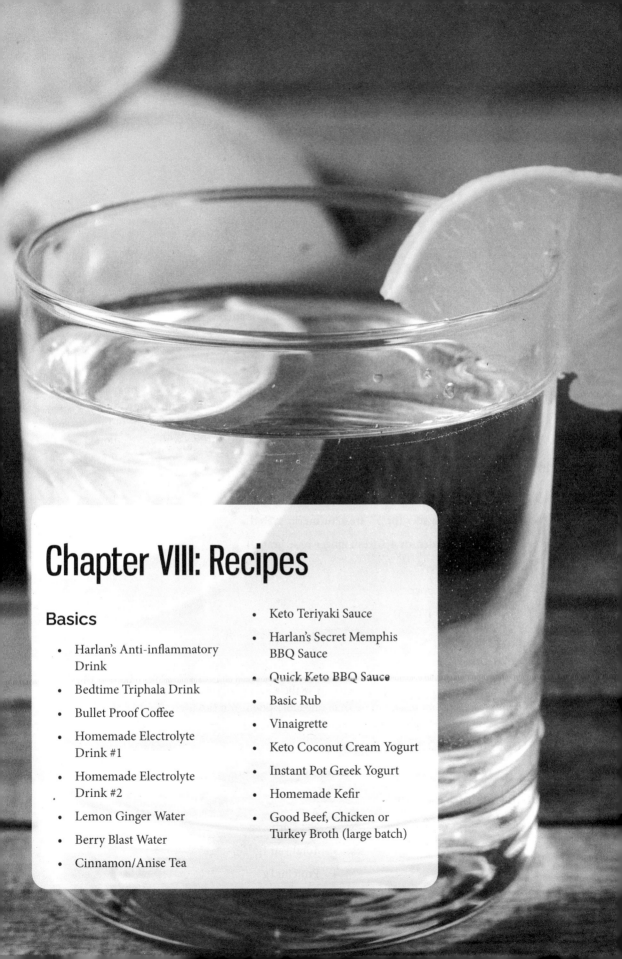

Chapter VIII: Recipes

Basics

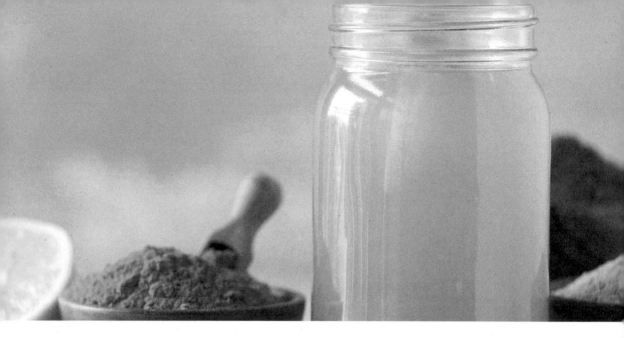

Harlan's Anti-inflammatory Drink

This recipe makes 1 drink so multiply ingredients by the number of people you are making drinks for this morning. It's easiest to simply line up the mugs and make the drinks individually. Freshly squeezed lemon juice is best as it has no extra additives to preserve the juice like the bottled version. One lemon usually yields ½ C of juice so you have enough for 2 drinks with each lemon.

Ingredients

- 3 T lemon juice, freshly squeezed
- 2 tsp turmeric powder (or 2 T fresh turmeric, grated)
- 4 tsp ginger powder (or 4 T fresh ginger root, grated)
- Dash black pepper
- Dash cayenne pepper
- 1 T Stevia (up to 1 Tbsp)
- ½ C water

Preparation

1. Mix all ingredients together in a glass. Use the stevia to sweeten the drink according to your own preference but use no more than one tablespoon. You can use either hot or cold water depending on your preference.

2. Drink only once a day, in the morning.

Yield: 1 Serving

Nutritional Information:

- Total Calories/Serving: 53
- Total Carbs: 10g
- Fiber: 2g
- Net Carbs: 8g
- Total Fat: 1g
- Protein: 1g

CompletelyKeto

Fat to Flat Master Plan: 28 Days To A Flat Tummy

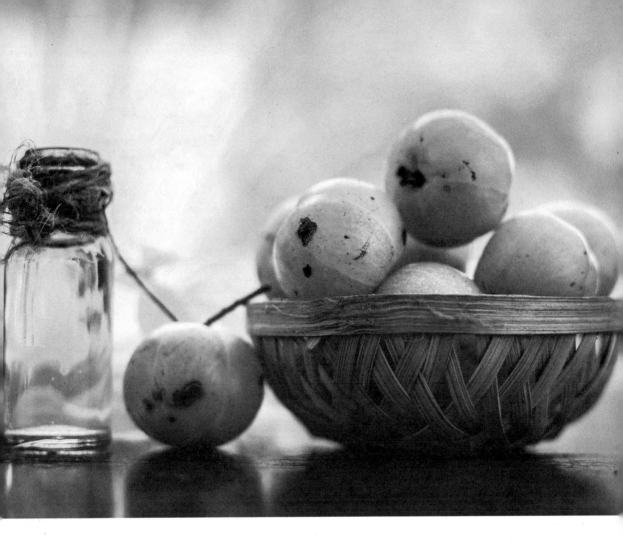

Bedtime Triphala Drink

Used for thousands of years in Ayurvedic medicine practice, Triphala is beneficial for digestion and elimination. It acts as a mild laxative and digestive tonic and stabilizes blood sugar. You can find it online.

Ingredients

- 1 tsp triphala
- ½ C hot or warm water
- 1 T fresh lemon or lime juice
- Stevia, to taste

Preparation

1. Stir 1 tsp of triphala into ½ C of either hot or warm water
2. Add 1 T of lemon or lime juice
3. Sweeten with liquid or powdered stevia, to taste. Drink on an empty stomach at bedtime.

Yield: 1 cup

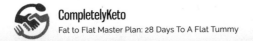

CompletelyKeto
Fat to Flat Master Plan: 28 Days To A Flat Tummy

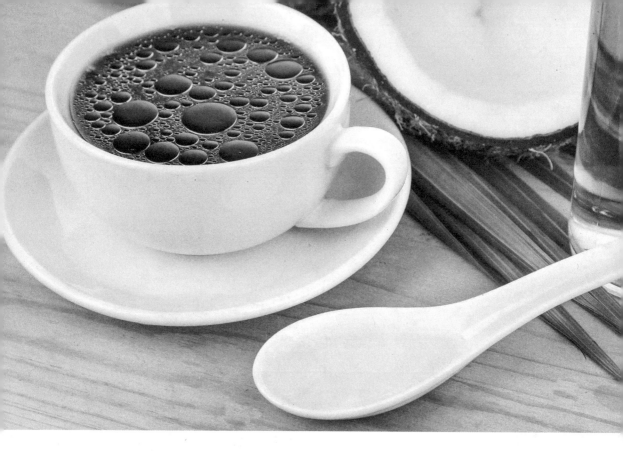

Bullet Proof Coffee

There are many different versions of bullet proof coffee out there on the internet. The Fat to Flat Masterplan version is simple:

- 1 cup of coffee with 1 tsp Brain Octane (MCT oil)

- That's it!

- Okay I hear the grumbling. You can have a teaspoon of ghee in your coffee. It's exactly like cream with the problems associated with dairy removed.

The usual time of day to drink this coffee is first thing in the morning because it immediately introduces an energy source for your body in the form of ketones. It`s just a great way to start the day. Only 2 Bullet Proof Coffees per day are allowed.

Note: Some people react with loose stools when first adding MCT oil to their diet. You will most likely be okay with just one teaspoon but if you notice a problem cut back to ½ tsp and slowly build up to 1 teaspoon in your bullet proof morning coffee.

Nutritional Information:

- Calories/serving: 45

- Total Carbs: 0

- Fiber: 0

- Total Fats: 5 g

- Protein: 0

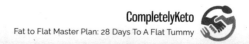

CompletelyKeto
Fat to Flat Master Plan: 28 Days To A Flat Tummy

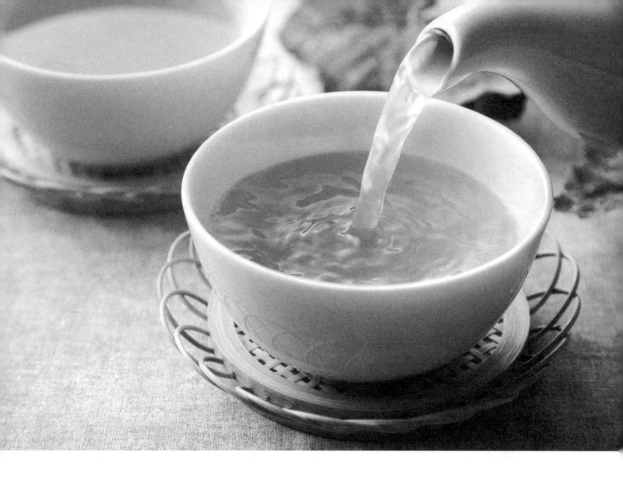

Homemade Electrolyte Drink #1

There are many brands of electrolyte drinks commercially available today but homemade is also a convenient and more economical option. You can pick up powdered magnesium supplement mixtures at most pharmacies, health food/supplement stores or you can also easily order it from online sources.

I use a fruit flavored herbal tea as a base for my homemade electrolyte brew and steep it with an added stevia leaf for sweetener. I know fresh stevia leaves aren't available to everyone so this recipe includes the option of sweetening to taste with the powdered or liquid version.

Ingredients

- 1 quart base liquid (green tea, flavored herbal tea, or plain water
- 1/8 -1/4 tsp pink Himalayan salt
- 1 tsp Calm (or other powdered magnesium supplement)
- Stevia sweetener (to taste)

Preparation

1. Brew tea if using, or slightly warm the base liquid.

2. Add Himalayan salt, magnesium powder and stevia (if using). Mix well until the additions have dissolved into the base liquid.

3. Store in refrigerator for up to four days.

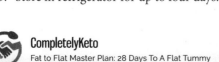

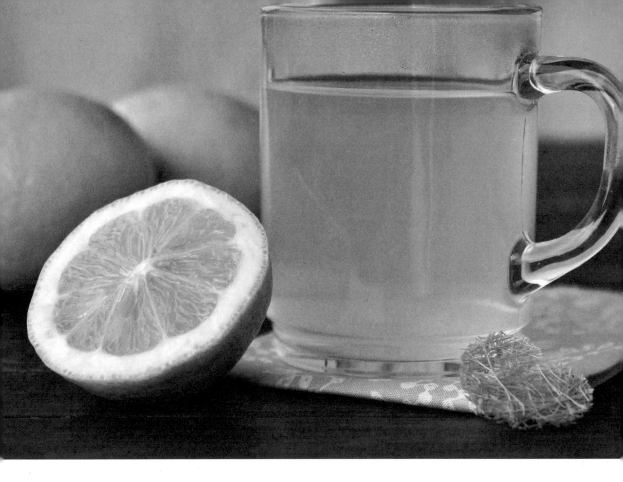

Homemade Electrolyte Drink #2

Ingredients

- ½ lemon, squeezed and seeds removed
- 1 T apple cider vinegar
- ¼ tsp No-Salt or Lo Salt
- ¼ tsp pink Himalayan salt
- 1 tsp Calm (or other magnesium supplement)
- Liquid stevia sweetener, to taste
- 2 cups water

Preparation

1. Combine all ingredients and enjoy!

Yield: 1 serving

Nutritional Information:

- Calories/serving: 10
- Net carbs: 2g
- Total Carbs: 2g
- Total Fat: 0g
- Fiber: 0g
- Protein: 0g

CompletelyKeto

Fat to Flat Master Plan: 28 Days To A Flat Tummy

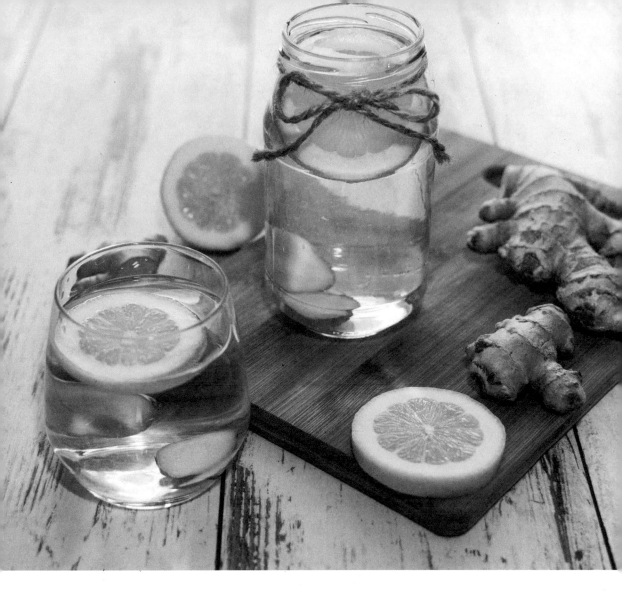

Lemon Ginger Water

The metabolic boost from ginger coupled with the detoxifying qualities of fresh lemon juice make this combo a treat for your whole digestive tract. Ginger is also known to calm an upset tummy and assists in taming acid reflux.

Ingredients

- 2" piece of ginger root, peeled
- 1 lemon, thinly sliced
- 6 C water
- Liquid stevia to taste, optional

Preparation

1. Place all ingredients in a glass container and cover with water.
2. Allow to rest, covered, for a few hours and room temperature and enjoy.

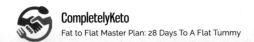

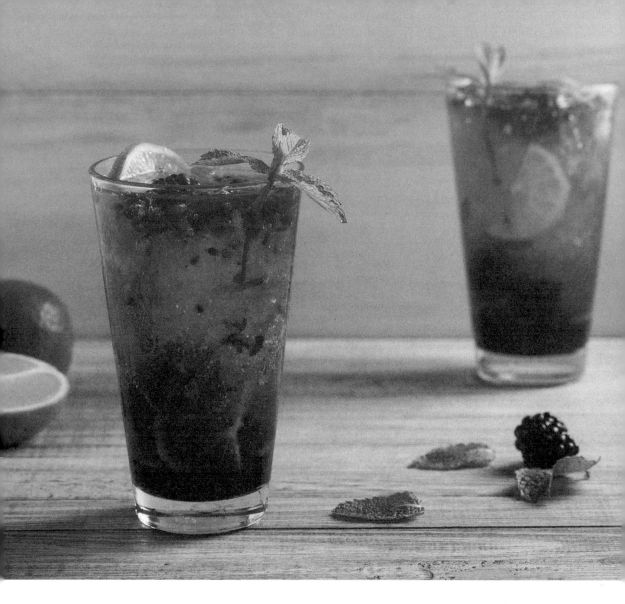

Berry Blast Water

Ingredients

- 1 C mixed berries (raspberries, blueberries, blackberries, strawberries)
- 1 lime, sliced thinly
- 1 lemon, sliced thinly
- Sprigs of fresh mint
- 8 C water
- Liquid stevia to taste, optional

Preparation

1. Place all ingredients in a glass container and cover with water.
2. Allow to rest, covered, for a few hours and room temperature and enjoy.

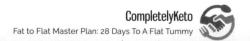

CompletelyKeto

Fat to Flat Master Plan: 28 Days To A Flat Tummy

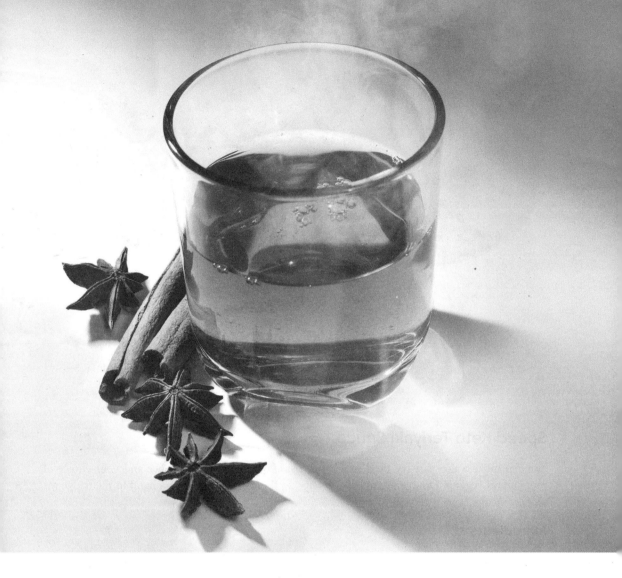

Cinnamon/Star Anise Tea

Cinnamon is known to help lower and maintain blood sugar levels by improving cell sensitivity to the action of the hormone insulin, which transports glucose from the blood into the cell to be used as energy.

Put this together with the antioxidant, anti-inflammatory and antimicrobial properties of star anise and you have a fine cup of tea to enjoy as often as you wish!

Ingredients

- 1 cinnamon stick
- 3 star anise pods
- 1-2 C boiling water

Preparation

1. Place all ingredients in a large mug and pour boiling water over-top. Allow tea to steep for 5-10 minutes and enjoy.

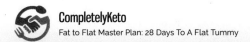

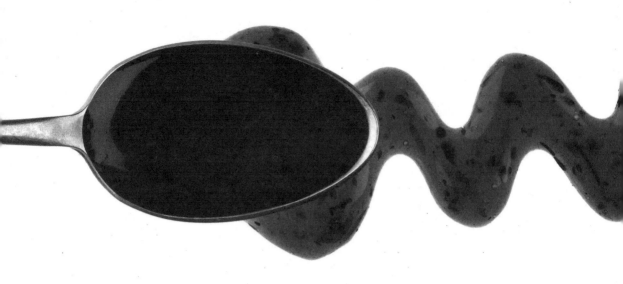

Speed Keto Teriyaki Sauce

You can make a nice stir-fry meal in a hurry using one batch of this sauce and your choice of protein and veggies. Double or triple this recipe so there's always some on hand in the fridge for an easy meal.

Ingredients

- ½ C gluten free tamari sauce
- Stevia (no more than 1 T), to taste
- 1 garlic clove, minced or pushed through a press
- 1 tsp ginger root, grated
- ½ C water
- ¼ tsp xanthan gum

Preparation

1. Whisk all ingredients and pour into a small saucepan. Heat over medium high heat while whisking until the sauce begins simmering and is thickened.

Yield: 4 servings (¼ C/serving)

Nutritional Information:

- Total Calories/Serving: 26
- Total Carbs: 3g
- Fiber: 1g
- Net Carbs: 2g
- Total Fat: 0g
- Protein: 4g

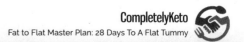

CompletelyKeto
Fat to Flat Master Plan: 28 Days To A Flat Tummy

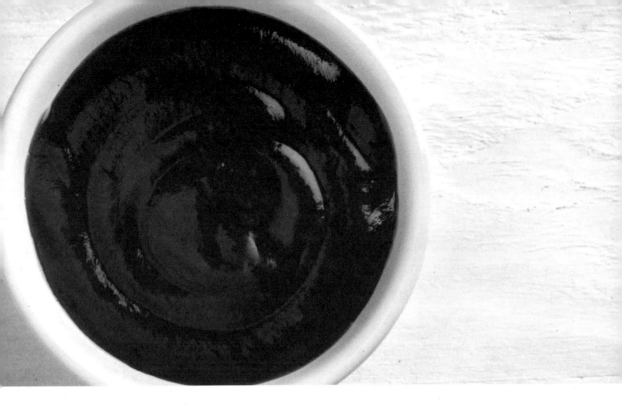

Harlan's Secret Memphis BBQ Sauce

Well I guess the secret is out! This tangy BBQ sauce adds extra flavor to many different dishes plus it's totally Keto. So fire up the BBQ and enjoy!

Ingredients

- 2 T coconut oil
- 1 medium onion, fine dice
- 2 cloves raw garlic, minced
- 2 T chili powder
- ½ tsp black pepper, ground
- ½ tsp cumin, ground
- ½ tsp oregano, dried
- 1 T basil, dried
- ¼ tsp sugar free liquid smoke
- 1 medium onion, fine dice
- 1 T deli style mustard
- 2 C marinara sauce, no sugar
- 2/3 C vinegar, apple cider
- ½ oz, bourbon
- 1 tsp hot sauce
- 2/3 C erythritol sweetener

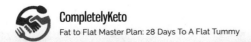

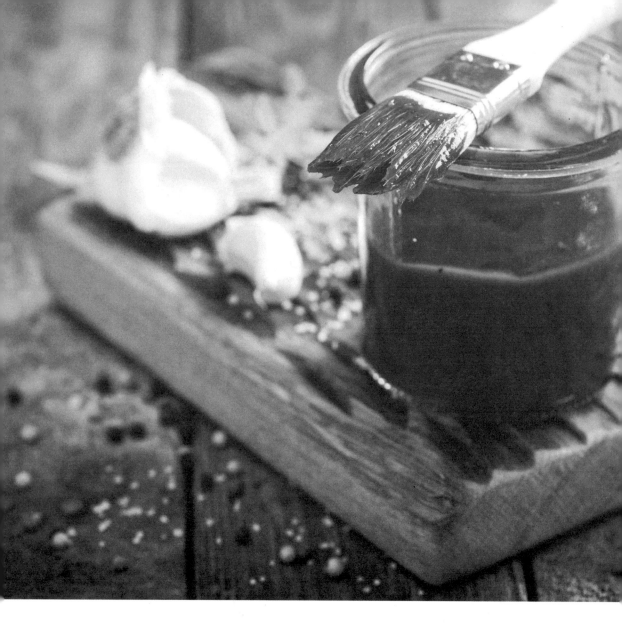

Preparation

1. Melt coconut oil in a stainless-steel pot, add diced onion and sauté for a few minutes until softened.

2. Add minced garlic, chili powder, pepper, cumin, oregano and basil. Continue to sauté for another few minutes.

3. Add remaining ingredients and simmer, stirring occasionally, for 20 minutes.

Yield: approximately 2 cups (2 T/serving)

Nutritional Information:

- Total Calories/serving: 41
- Net Carbs: 3g
- Total Carbs :4g
- Total Fat: 3g
- Fiber: 1g
- Protein: 1g

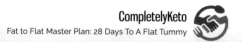

CompletelyKeto
Fat to Flat Master Plan: 28 Days To A Flat Tummy

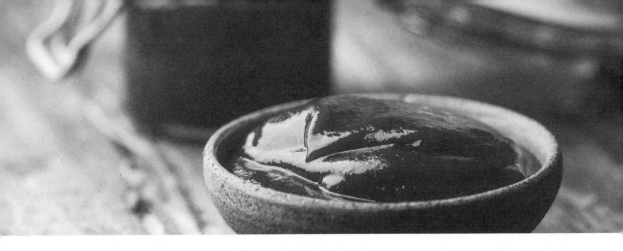

Quick Keto BBQ Sauce

This BBQ sauce whisks together quickly and after a short simmering process you are done.

Ingredients

- ¾ C no sugar added ketchup
- ½ C water
- ¼ C vinegar, white or apple cider
- 2 tsp garlic granules
- 2 tsp onion powder
- 1 T chili powder
- ½ tsp dried oregano
- ¼ tsp ground cumin
- 1 tsp smoked chipotle powder
- 1 tsp smoked paprika
- Grinding of black peppercorns
- Approved sweetener (to taste)

Preparation

1. Place all ingredients in a small, heavy bottomed saucepan and whisk together. Turn the heat under the pot up to medium high until the sauce comes to a boil then lower the heat, so the mixture is just simmering. Simmer for 10 minutes while stirring occasionally.

2. Remove from heat and allow sauce to cool down before storing in an air-tight container in the fridge.

Yield: 20 Servings (1 T/serving)

Nutritional Information:

- Calories/serving: 10
- Net Carbs: 1g
- Total Carbs: 1g
- Total Fat: 0g
- Fiber: 0g
- Protein:

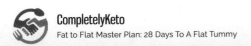

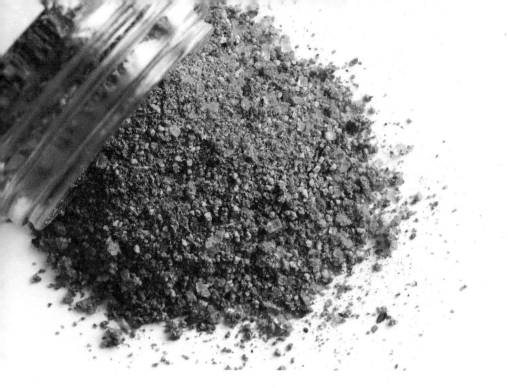

Basic Rub

This is my go-to rub when it's time for BBQ. I use it on beef, chicken and turkey.

Ingredients

- 2 T granulated garlic
- 2 T onion powder
- ½ T chili powder
- 1 tsp smoked chipotle powder
- 1 tsp smoked paprika
- 2 tsp oregano
- ½ T salt flakes
- 2 T erythritol/stevia mix (or approved sweetener of your choice)

Preparation

1. Stir all ingredients together until well combined.
2. Store at room temperature in an air-tight container.

Yield: 16 Servings (1 T/serving)

Nutritional Information:

- Calories/serving: 7
- Total Carbs: 2g
- Fiber: 2g
- Net Carbs: 0g
- Total Fat: 1g
- Protein: 0g

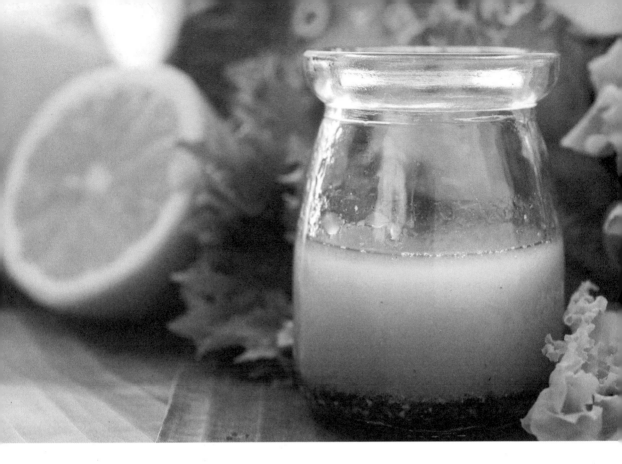

Vinaigrette

Homemade vinaigrettes are easy to make. Once you get onto how easy it is to whip one up there will be no going back to heavy handed, fake tasting store bought salad dressings.

Ingredients

- Juice from 1 lemon or 2 limes
- 1 tsp Dijon mustard
- 3 drops of liquid stevia
- ¾ C olive oil

Preparation

1. Whisk lemon juice, mustard and liquid stevia.
2. Drizzle olive oil into the lemon juice mixture and continue whisking until all the oil has been incorporated into the dressing.

Yield: 16 servings (1 Tablespoon in each serving)

Nutritional Information:

- Total Calories/serving: 90
- Net Carbs: 0g
- Total Carbs: 0g
- Total Fat: 10 g
- Fiber: 0g
- Protein: 0 g

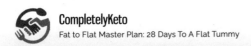

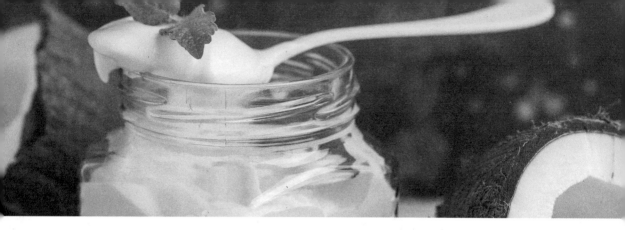

Keto Coconut Cream Yogurt

I've used the powder from probiotic capsules to culture the yogurt in this recipe but you could also purchase a packet of powder that's been specifically created for use in the process of making yogurt at home. Yogurt made from this way may be a bit mellower than the tangy tasting yogurt you get when using probiotic capsules.

Note: When making your next batch of yogurt you can simply use 3 tsp. of yogurt from this batch as the culture in your next batch.

Ingredients

- 2 cans (400 ml/ 13.5 oz) full-fat coconut cream, use thick part (coconut cream) only
- 2 mixed strain probiotics capsules (or ¾ tsp of probiotic powder)
- Liquid stevia to taste, optional
- Vanilla to taste, optional

Preparation

1. Refrigerate coconut cream in cans overnight. This will allow the coconut cream to separate from the small amount of coconut water in the cans. It will harden at the top of the can.

2. Open the cans and spoon out the hardened cream. Place the cream in a clean and sterilized mason jar. Stir in 3 T of the coconut water.

3. Carefully pull apart the probiotics capsules and empty the contents into the mason jar. Stir and then cover the jar by tying on a few layers of cheesecloth. The cheesecloth will allow some air to flow through while the yogurt ferments. Store in a dark, room temperature cupboard, for 24 – 48 hours. If it's warm it will only take about 24 hours for the yogurt to thicken but if it is cooler it take the full 48 hours (and perhaps even a bit longer).

4. When done, seal the jar with a lid and refrigerate for up to 4 days. The yogurt will thicken a bit more in the colder fridge. You can sweeten the yogurt with liquid stevia, if desired.

Yield: 6 Servings (about ½ C/serving)

Nutritional Information:

- Calories/serving: 220
- Total Carbs: 3g
- Fiber: 1g

- Net carbs: 2g
- Total Fat: 23g
- Protein: 1g

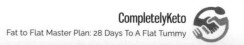

CompletelyKeto
Fat to Flat Master Plan: 28 Days To A Flat Tummy

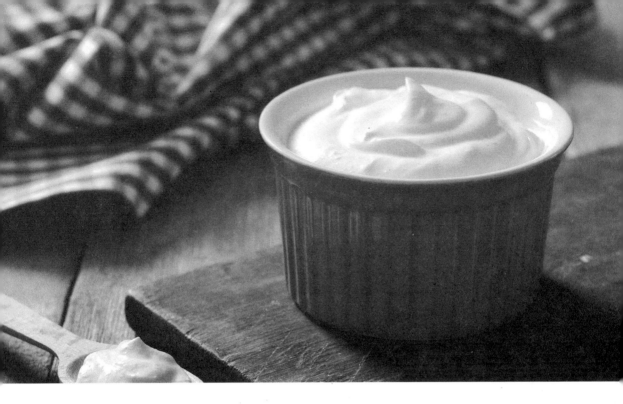

Instant Pot Greek Yogurt

Ingredients

- 2 C whole milk
- 2 C heavy cream
- 2 T Greek (live culture) yogurt or (powder from 2 probiotic capsules or packet of yogurt starter culture powder)

Preparation

1. Pour milk and cream into instant pot and seal lid. Program the "keep warm" setting for 40 minutes. Remove lid, change setting to sauté and whisk while the milk mixture warms up to 180 F. T

2. Take the liner from the instant pot and allow the milk mixture to rest as it cools to 110 F. Unplug the instant pot.

3. Whisk yogurt (or powdered culture) into cooled milk. Place the liner back into the instant pot (leave the pot unplugged).

4. Seal the lid and leave the pot alone for 8 hours. You should have a nice thick and creamy Greek yogurt when you open the lid. Store refrigerated, in a glass jar, for up to one week.

Yield: 8 Servings (1/2 C/serving)

Nutritional Information:

- Calories/serving: 53
- Net carbs: 3g
- Total Carbs: 3g
- Total Fat: 4g
- Fiber: 0g
- Protein: 2g

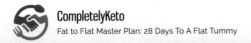

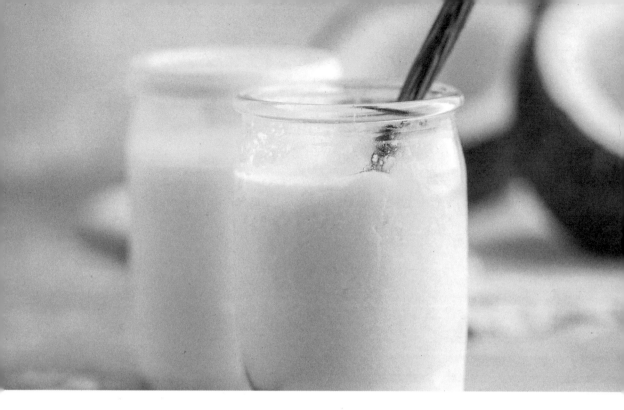

Homemade Kefir

My version of kefir is made with coconut milk and has only 4g net carbs per serving!

Ingredients

- 4 C full fat coconut milk
- 1 packet of kefir starter culture
- ¼ tsp pure vanilla
- Liquid stevia, to taste

Preparation

1. Pour full fat coconut milk into 1 quart mason jar. Add the kefir starter culture grains and seal the jar. Give it a good shake to mix the grains with the milk then place the jar in a warm place (72F - 85F). Leave for 24-48 hours. I place mine in the oven with the oven light turned on.

2. Do a taste-test after 24 hours. If it isn't done to your taste, leave it to ferment for (up to) another 24 hours. When done give the jar a shake and refrigerate. Use within 5 days.

Yield: 4 Servings (1 C/serving)

Nutritional Information:

- Calories/serving: 50
- Net carbs: 4g
- Total Carbs: 4g
- Total Fat: 5g
- Fiber: 0g
- Protein: 1g

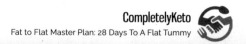

CompletelyKeto
Fat to Flat Master Plan: 28 Days To A Flat Tummy

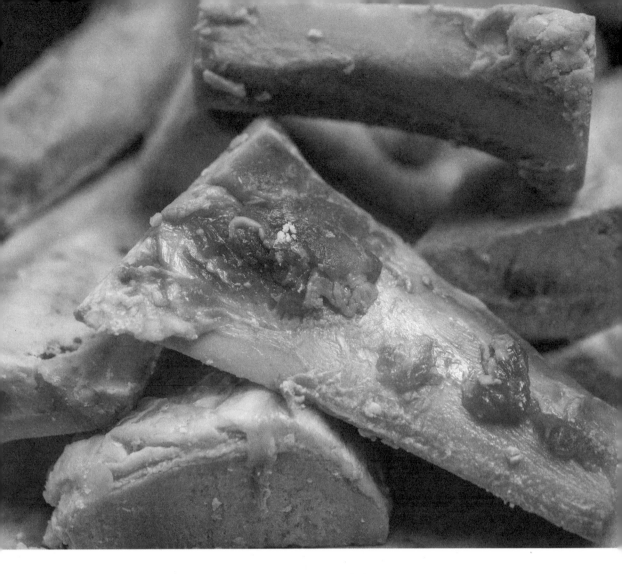

Good Beef, Chicken or Turkey Bone Broth (large batch)

Make this recipe for bone broth on the weekend. It can be simmering on the stove or in an instant pot or large crock pot while you are home doing chores. Bone Broth is a staple in our fridge. We use it as the base for different nutritious soups or for a simple and satisfying drink during intermittent fasting. If I find myself hungry between meals (which isn't very often), I opt to sip on a cup of homemade bone broth. I freeze bone broth in ice cube trays for this purpose. When the broth is frozen I simply store cubes in a re-sealable plastic bag for use as needed.

You can also save your chicken or turkey carcasses in the freezer and make a fine bone broth from them when you have time. Use at least three small carcasses when making chicken bone broth. I also opt to use a whole chicken if I don't have any chicken carcasses handy. When I do this I simply simmer the whole chicken, covered with water and the other ingredients until the meat reaches an internal temperature of 165 F. I then remove the chicken from the pot and take the meat from the bones and return the bones and skin to the pot and let it simmer for a few more hours. The chicken meat can be cooled and frozen for use in recipes as the week progresses.

A turkey carcass will work well too. Follow the recipe below, omitting the first 2 steps if making chicken or turkey bone broth.

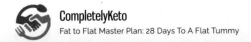

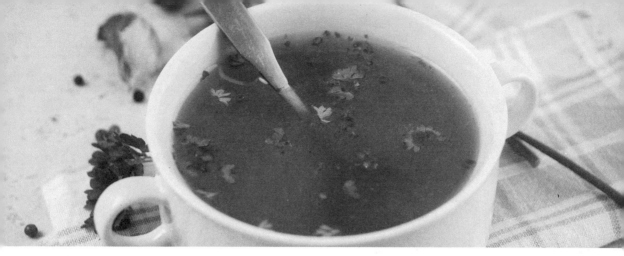

Ingredients

- 6 beef marrow bone chunks (2 -2½ lb) (or two small chicken carcasses)
- Water (to cover bones)
- 2 T apple cider vinegar
- 10 pepper corns
- 1 bay leaf
- ½ bunch of fresh flat or curly leaf parsley (or 1 T dried parsley)
- Sprig of fresh thyme (½ tsp dried)
- Sprig of fresh rosemary (½ tsp ground)
- ¾ tsp ground Himalayan salt

Preparation

1. Pre-heat oven to 375 F

2. Put beef bones on a rimmed pan lined with foil. Place the pan on the middle rack of the pre-heated oven and roast the bones for 1 hour. Be careful when removing the pan from the oven as there will be some melted fat in the bottom of the shallow pan that will be very hot. Skip if using chicken carcasses.

3. Stove-top method: Place the roasted bones (or chicken carcasses) and any melted fat in a large stock pot and add the cider vinegar and water. Allow bones (carcasses) to soak for 20 minutes before adding the remaining ingredients. Bring to a boil and then reduce the heat under the pot so the broth is just simmering. Place the pot lid on top so it's slightly askew to allow steam to escape as the broth simmers. Skim the top of the liquid every 20 minutes or so during the first 1 ½ hours. You may need to add more water now and then, depending on how long you simmer the bone broth. We suggest at least 3 – 4 hours. When it's done remove from heat and let cool for a while before removing the bones then strain the broth through a large sized sieve. Discard the mushy vegetables and bones. Store the bone broth marked for use over the next few days in the fridge and freeze the remainder.

4. Instant Pot Method: Place roasted bones (chicken carcasses) and any melted fat into a 6 quart instant pot. Add remaining ingredients and cover with water (fill up to 1" below the highest mark in your pot).

Yield: Approximately 10 servings, 1 C each

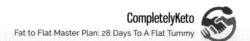

CompletelyKeto
Fat to Flat Master Plan: 28 Days To A Flat Tummy

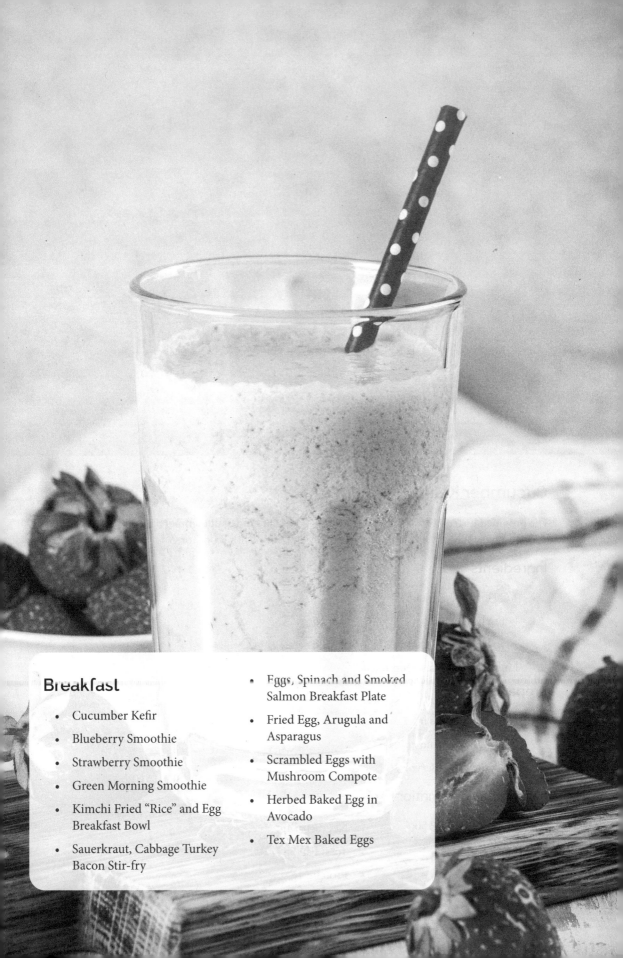

Breakfast

- Cucumber Kefir
- Blueberry Smoothie
- Strawberry Smoothie
- Green Morning Smoothie
- Kimchi Fried "Rice" and Egg Breakfast Bowl
- Sauerkraut, Cabbage Turkey Bacon Stir-fry
- Eggs, Spinach and Smoked Salmon Breakfast Plate
- Fried Egg, Arugula and Asparagus
- Scrambled Eggs with Mushroom Compote
- Herbed Baked Egg in Avocado
- Tex Mex Baked Eggs

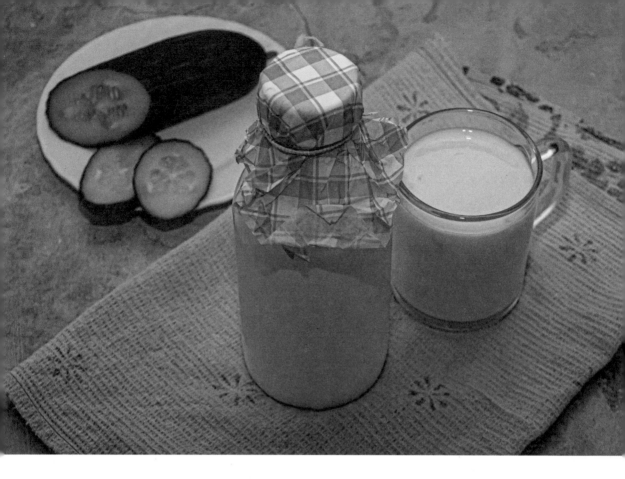

Cucumber Kefir

I've provided instructions for making your own kefir at home but commercial kefir, made without added sugars is readily available at the grocery store or health food store.

Ingredients

- 1 C Homemade Kefir
- ½ English cucumber
- 2 tsp chopped fresh mint (or 1 tsp dried mint)
- Liquid stevia to taste, optional

Preparation

1. Place ingredients in high speed blender and process until smooth.
2. Pour into glass and enjoy!

Yield: 4 Servings (1 C/serving)

Nutritional Information:

- Calories/serving: 50
- Total Carbs: 4g
- Fiber: 0g
- Net carbs: 4g
- Total Fat: 5g
- Protein: 1g

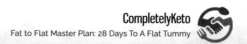

CompletelyKeto

Fat to Flat Master Plan: 28 Days To A Flat Tummy

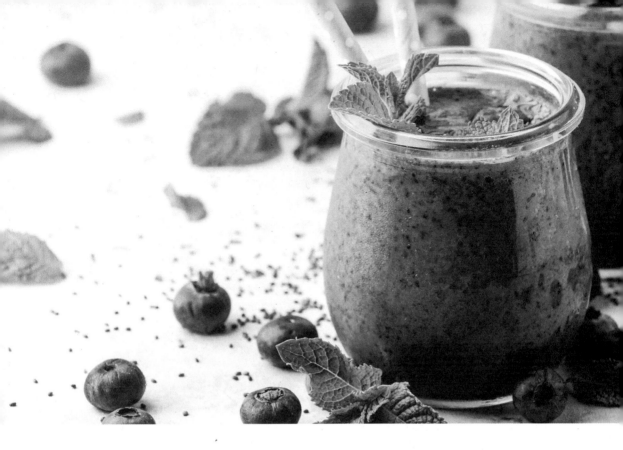

Blueberry Smoothie

Ingredients

- 1/3 C frozen blueberries
- ½ C Homemade Instant Pot Greek Yogurt or ½ C Keto Coconut Cream Yogurt
- ¼ C water
- Liquid stevia to taste, optional

Preparation

1. Process all ingredients in blender until smooth and enjoy.

Yield: 1 Serving

Nutritional Information:

made with Keto Coconut Cream Yogurt

- Calories/serving: 248
- Total Carbs: 10g
- Fiber: 2g
- Net carbs: 8g
- Total Fat: 23g
- Protein: 1g

Nutritional Information:

made with Instant Pot Greek Yogurt

- Calories/serving: 81
- Total Carbs: 10g
- Fiber: 1g
- Net carbs: 7g
- Total Fat: 6g
- Protein: 3g

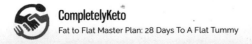

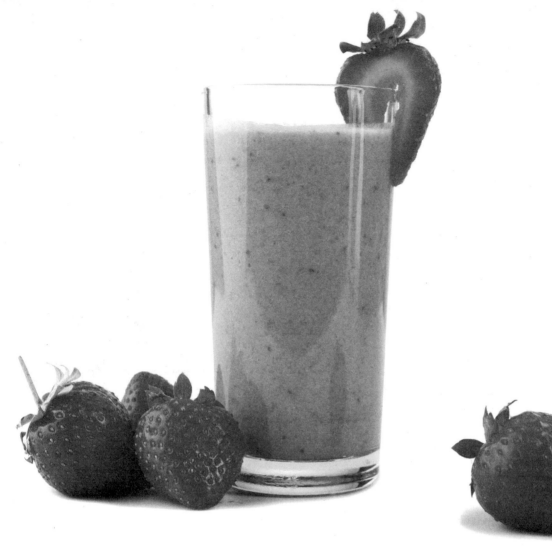

Strawberry Smoothie

Ingredients

- ½ C frozen strawberries
- ¼ C water
- ½ C Instant Pot Greek Yogurt
- Liquid stevia to taste, optional

Preparation

1. Process all ingredients in blender until smooth and enjoy.

Yield: 1 Serving

Nutritional Information:

- Calories/serving: 80
- Net carbs: 7g
- Total Carbs: 9
- Total Fat: 4g
- Fiber: 2g
- Protein: 3g

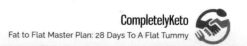

CompletelyKeto
Fat to Flat Master Plan: 28 Days To A Flat Tummy

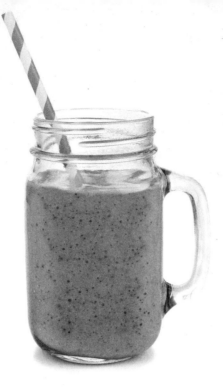

Green Morning Smoothie

Start your day with this green smoothie. The bright taste of mint and splash of tangy lime juice brightens the flavor plus the fat from the avocado will give you some get up and go energy.

Ingredients

- ½ Hass avocado
- 3 mint leaves
- ¼ C cilantro leaves
- 1 T fresh lime juice
- ½ C full fat coconut milk
- ¼ C water
- ¼ tsp pure vanilla
- Liquid stevia to taste, optional

Preparation

1. Place all ingredients into a high speed blender and process until the ice is crushed and the texture is smooth.

Yield: 1 Serving

Nutritional Information:

- Calories/serving: 346
- Total Carbs: 11g
- Fiber: 6g
- Net carbs: 5g
- Total Fat: 32g
- Protein: 3g

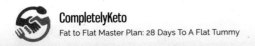

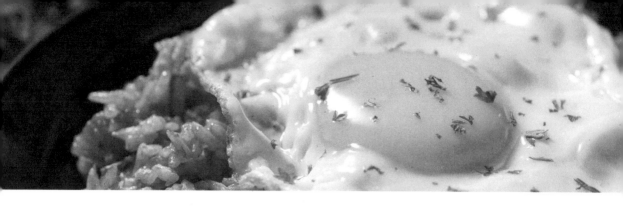

Kimchi Fried "Rice" and Egg Breakfast Bowl

Ready in 15 minutes, this keto breakfast provides a good start to the day with flavor that packs a punch!

Ingredients

- 5 C cauliflower florets (or use 4 C frozen cauliflower rice)
- 2 T plus 1 T extra-virgin olive oil, divided
- 2/3 C Keto Kimchi
- 2 garlic cloves, minced or pushed through a press
- 1 T fresh ginger root, minced
- 2 T kimchi juice
- 1 T gluten free tamari sauce
- Grinding of pink Himalayan salt and black peppercorns, to taste
- 4 eggs

Preparation

1. Place cauliflower florets in high speed blender (or food processor) and pulse a few times until florets are cut into rice-sized bits.

2. Heat 2 T of the oil in a wok over medium high heat. Add the cauliflower rice, kimchi, garlic, kimchi juice and tamari sauce. Stir-fry for about 5 minutes until the cauliflower rice softens and is cooked and the kimchi is heated through. Season mixture with a grinding of salt and pepper. Set aside and keep warm.

3. Heat remaining oil in a heavy bottomed skillet over medium high heat. Fry eggs to your liking.

4. Divide cauliflower rice/kimchi mixture between 4 bowls and top each with a fried egg. Serve immediately.

Yield: 4 Servings

Nutritional Information:

- Calories/serving: 242
- Net carbs: 6
- Total Carbs: 12
- Total Fat: 15g
- Fiber: 6
- Protein: 12g

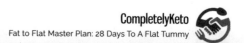

CompletelyKeto
Fat to Flat Master Plan: 28 Days To A Flat Tummy

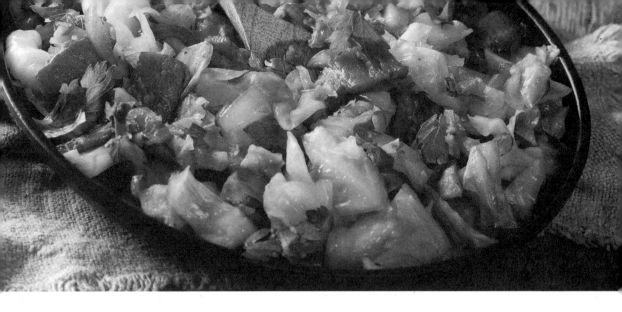

Sauerkraut, Cabbage and Turkey Bacon Stir-fry

This simple stir-fry makes quick lunch on its own or a perfect side-dish at dinner time. We like the added tang of sauerkraut in this easy to prepare recipe.

Ingredients

- 1 T plus ½ T extra-virgin olive oil
- ¼ C cooking onion, small dice
- 2 C cabbage, shredded
- 2 C sauerkraut
- 4 strips thick-cut turkey bacon
- 4 eggs

Preparation

1. Heat oil in a wok or heavy bottomed skillet over medium high heat. Add diced onion and stir-fry for a few minutes until the onion is softened and translucent.

2. Add the cabbage and stir-fry for 4 or 5 minutes until the cabbage is wilted and cooked. Add the sauerkraut and stir-fry until everything is heated through. Toss in the prepared bacon and stir-fry for one more minute. Remove from heat and keep warm.

3. Heat remaining oil in a heavy bottomed skillet. Fry eggs to your liking.

4. Divide cabbage/sauerkraut mixture between 4 bowls and top each with a fried egg. Serve immediately.

Yield: 4 Servings

Nutritional Information:

- Calories/serving: 197
- Total Carbs: 8g
- Fiber: 1g
- Net carbs: 7g
- Total Fat: 13g
- Protein: 13g

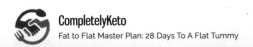

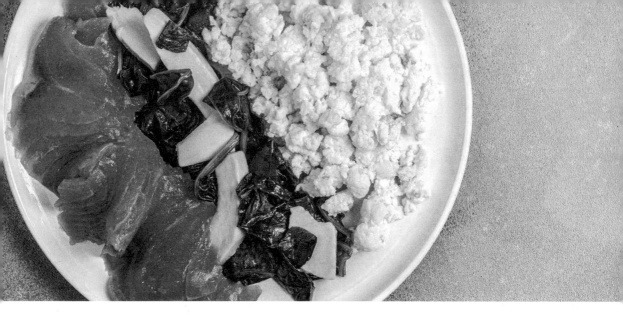

Eggs, Spinach and Smoked Salmon Breakfast Plate

Here is another low carb breakfast which provides a nutritious start to a busy day. Smoked salmon is a staple in our house that we often turn to for easy protein and maximum flavor when time is at a minimum.

Ingredients

- 12 oz smoked salmon, thin slices
- 1 T extra-virgin olive oil
- 1 garlic clove
- 4 C baby spinach leaves
- ½ ripe avocado, peeled and cut into slices
- Grinding of pink Himalayan salt and black peppercorns
- 6 eggs, whisked

Preparation

1. Arrange salmon on 4 plates. Set aside.

2. Heat ½ T of the oil in a heavy bottomed skillet. Add baby spinach and garlic. Sauté for a few minutes until the spinach wilts and is heated through. Season with a quick grinding of salt and pepper. Divide evenly amongst the plates

3. Heat remaining oil in the same skillet and scramble the whisked eggs to your liking. Season, divide the eggs and avocado slices amongst the plates and serve immediately.

Yield: 4 servings

Nutritional Information:

- Calories/serving: 320
- Net carbs: 2g
- Total Carbs: 3g
- Total Fat: 20g
- Fiber: 1g
- Protein: 32g

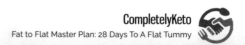

CompletelyKeto

Fat to Flat Master Plan: 28 Days To A Flat Tummy

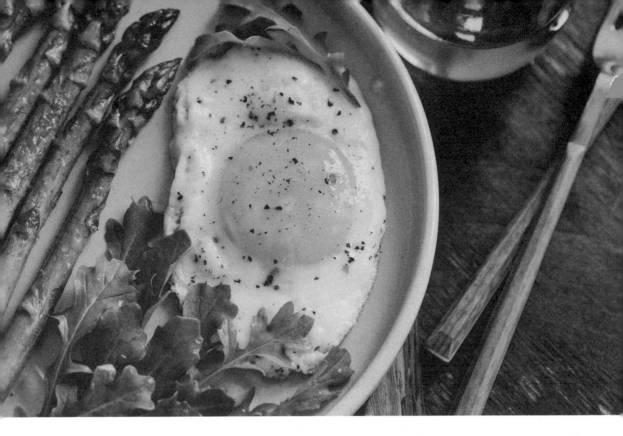

Fried Egg, Arugula and Asparagus Breakfast Plate

This combination of veggie, greens and eggs always pleases at breakfast time; plus, it just looks plain pretty on the plate!

Ingredients

- 16 asparagus spears, trimmed
- 2 tsp extra virgin olive oil
- 4 eggs
- 1 C arugula

Preparation

1. Steam asparagus over boiling water for 4 minutes.
2. While asparagus is cooking heat oil in heavy bottomed skillet over medium high heat. Fry or poach eggs to your liking.
3. Divide asparagus, arugula and fried eggs between 4 plates. Serve and enjoy.

Yield: 4 Servings

Nutritional Information:

- Calories/serving: 100
- Total Carbs: 1g
- Fiber: 0g
- Net carbs: 1g
- Total Fat: 8g
- Protein: 7g

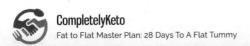

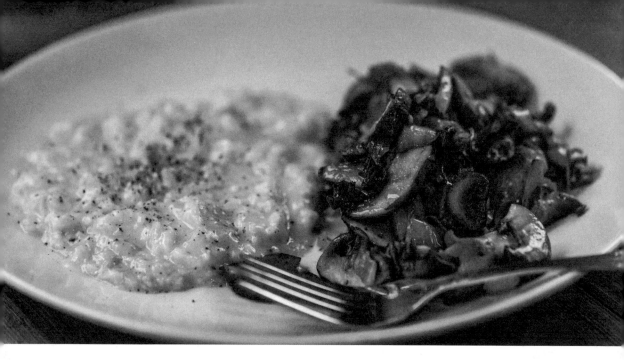

Scrambled Eggs with Mushroom Compote

This is an easy and nourishing breakfast to start your day. Scrambled eggs are one of my go-to comfort foods in the morning.

Ingredients

- 1 T extra-virgin olive oil
- ½ lb cremini mushrooms, sliced
- ½ C baby spinach leaves
- 4 eggs, whisked
- Grinding of pink Himalayan salt and black peppercorns

Preparation

1. Heat half of the oil in a heavy bottomed skillet over medium high heat. Add mushrooms and sauté until mushrooms are done and most of the moisture has evaporated from the pan.

2. Stir in the spinach and stir until it wilts. Season to taste with a quick grinding of salt and pepper, remove from pan and keep warm. Wipe out pan, add remaining oil and return to the heat.

3. Pour eggs into the pan when the oil is hot and scramble until done to your liking and correct the seasoning. Divide mushroom compote and eggs between two plates and serve.

Yield: 4 servings

Nutritional Information:

- Calories/serving: 131
- Net carbs: 2.3g
- Total Carbs: 3.3g
- Total Fat: 8.9g
- Fiber: 1g
- Protein: 8.4g

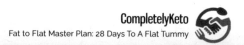
CompletelyKeto
Fat to Flat Master Plan: 28 Days To A Flat Tummy

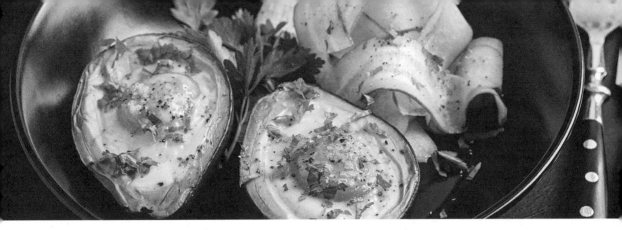

Herbed Baked Egg in Avocado

There are a variety of additions that can be tucked in with egg in that lovely little hollow inside the avocado; various herbs, smoked salmon, small ham cubes and turkey sausage or turkey bacon bits all can add flavor to this easy meal.

Today I'm choosing smoked herbs for this recipe but you could easily let your family customize their own avocado baked avocado egg dish. I like serving Garlic Zucchini Noodles if I'm making this for lunch or dinner.

Ingredients

- 2 T mixed fresh herbs
- 1 ripe Hass avocado, cut in half and pit removed
- 2 eggs
- Grinding of pink Himalayan salt and black peppercorns
- Fresh snipped herbs for garnish, if desired

Preparation

1. Pre-heat oven to 350 F.
2. Cut avocado in half and remove pit. Leave skin on. Hollow out the interior a bit so there's room enough inside the boat to hold the egg.
3. Place 2 T of freshly snipped herbs inside the hollow.
4. Crack an egg into the cavity of one of the avocado halves and season with salt and pepper. Place avocado boat on a parchment-lined, rimmed baking sheet. Do the same with the second avocado half.
5. Place baking sheet on the middle rack of the pre-heated oven for 20-25 minutes or until the eggs are done to your liking. Garnish with herbs, if desired and serve immediately.

Yield: 2 Servings

Nutritional Information:

- Total Calories/Serving: 284
- Total Carbs: 6g
- Fiber: 5g
- Net Carbs: 1g
- Total Fat: 22g
- Protein: 18g

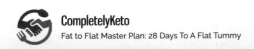

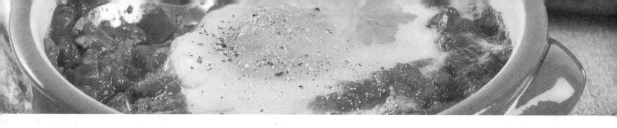

Tex Mex Baked Eggs

Baked eggs nestled into spiced ground meat make a fine presentation when brought to the table straight from the oven. Great for a brunch; but easy enough to pull together for a week day breakfast, lunch or dinner when time is at a premium.

Ingredients

- 1 lb ground beef, ground pork, ground turkey or ground chicken
- 2 garlic cloves, minced or pushed through a press
- ¼ C red pepper, small dice
- ¼ tsp smoked chipotle powder
- ½ tsp chili powder
- ½ tsp garlic powder
- ½ tsp onion powder
- ¼ C tomato sauce, no sugar
- ¼ C beef broth
- 3 eggs
- Fermented Hot Sauce or Fermented Red Salsa for garnish, if desired

Preparation

1. Pre-heat oven to 375F.

2. Heat a heavy bottomed, oven proof skillet over high heat and add ground meat, and spices. Lower heat to medium high and sauté the meat while stirring until it's partially cooked.

3. Add garlic cloves and continue to sauté until the meat is browned and almost done. Add the tomato sauce and broth and simmer the mixture until the sauce thickens and the meat is cooked through (about 5 minute). Correct the seasoning with salt and pepper. Divide between three small casserole dishes.

4. Make three wells in the meat mixture and crack an egg into each well. Place on the middle rack of the pre-heated oven and bake 10-15 minutes or until the eggs are done to your liking. Let sit for a few minutes before serving.

5. Garnish with a few tablespoons of Fermented Hot Sauce or Fermented Red Salsa, if desired.

Yield: 3 Servings

Nutritional Information:

- Total Calories/Serving: 360
- Total Carbs: 4g
- Fiber: 1g
- Total Fat: 21g
- Protein: 38g

CompletelyKeto
Fat to Flat Master Plan: 28 Days To A Flat Tummy

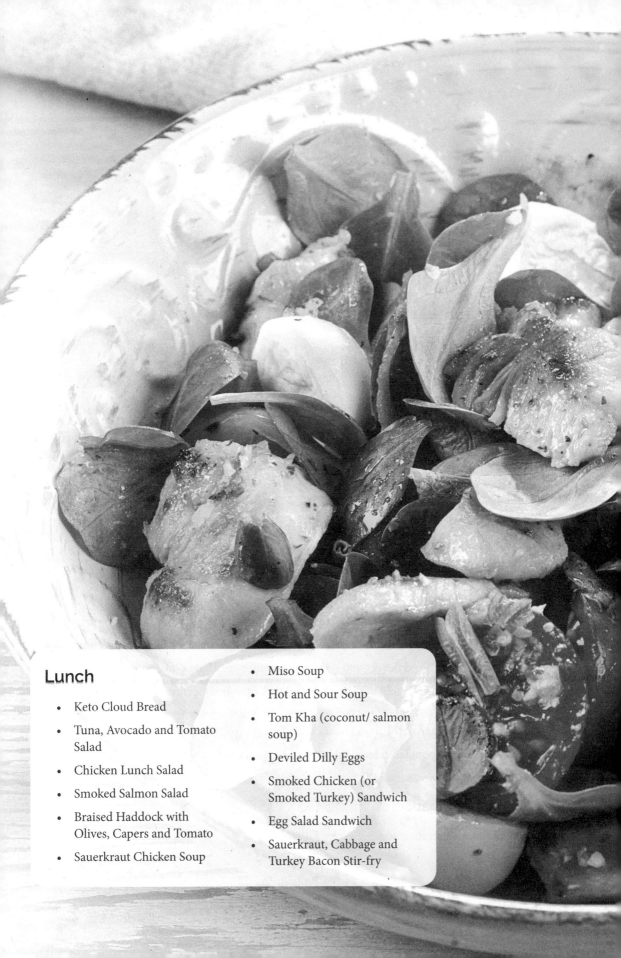

Lunch

- Keto Cloud Bread
- Tuna, Avocado and Tomato Salad
- Chicken Lunch Salad
- Smoked Salmon Salad
- Braised Haddock with Olives, Capers and Tomato
- Sauerkraut Chicken Soup
- Miso Soup
- Hot and Sour Soup
- Tom Kha (coconut/ salmon soup)
- Deviled Dilly Eggs
- Smoked Chicken (or Smoked Turkey) Sandwich
- Egg Salad Sandwich
- Sauerkraut, Cabbage and Turkey Bacon Stir-fry

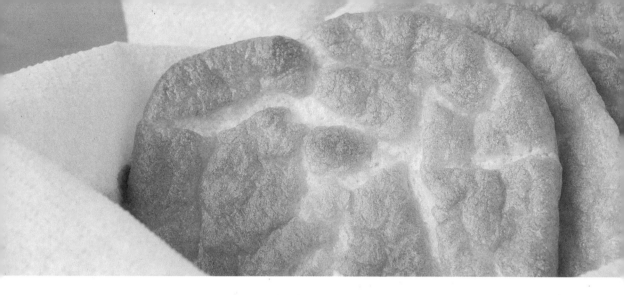

Keto Cloud Bread

This bread keeps well in the fridge for three days. If you freeze it make sure to slip a piece of parchment paper between the slices so they won't stick together. It's a good idea to always have this cloud bread available for a quick lunch sandwich.

Recipes for Cloud bread are all over the internet with no one really being clear about where it originated. Most of these recipes use cream cheese instead of mayo. Here's our favorite version. We love it because the ingredients are compatible with food allowed on all my versions of Speed Keto.

Ingredients

- 3 large eggs, separated
- 1/8 tsp cream of tartar
- 3 T Keto Mayonnaise, no sugar

Preparation

1. Pre-heat oven to 300 F.
2. Whip egg white with a hand held mixer until they thicken slightly.
3. Sprinkle the cream of tartar over the whites and continue to whip until stiff peaks form.
4. Using the mixer blend the egg yolks and mayonnaises until light and creamy.
5. Using a spatula, gently fold the egg white and yolk mixtures together to form a batter.
6. Make 6 separate mounds of the batter on a parchment lined baking sheet, leaving a bit of space between each of the round pancake shapes.
7. Bake until lightly golden colored (about 30 minutes). Cool on a wire rack.

Yield: 6 servings (one piece/serving)

Nutritional Information:

- Total Calories/serving: 86
- Total Carbs: 0g
- Fiber: 0g
- Total Fat: 8g
- Protein: 3g

CompletelyKeto
Fat to Flat Master Plan: 28 Days To A Flat Tummy

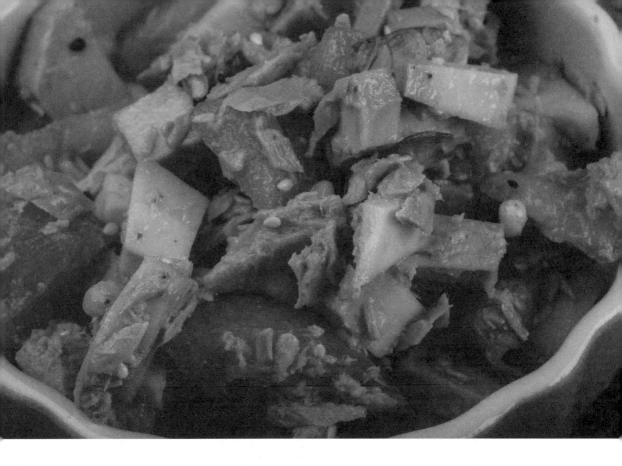

Tuna, Avocado and Tomato Salad

Canned tuna is always available in my pantry because it's a versatile protein. This a go-to lunch salad recipe when I have ripe avocados in my kitchen. Pair the salad with fermented veggies of choice and lunch is prepared in just a few minutes.

Ingredients

- 2 cans solid Tuna, drained and pulled apart into bite-sized chunks
- 2 medium tomatoes, medium dice
- 2 ripe Hass avocado, seeded, peeled and cut into bite-sized chunks
- 2 tsp dried dill (or 2 T fresh dill leaves)
- 2 T vinaigrette or other approved dressing of choice

Preparation

1. Combine all ingredients, toss, divide between 4 salad bowls and serve.

Yield: 4 Servings

Nutritional Information:

- Calories/serving: 274
- Net carbs: 4g
- Total Carbs: 12g
- Total Fat: 22g
- Fiber: 8g
- Protein: 11g

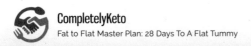

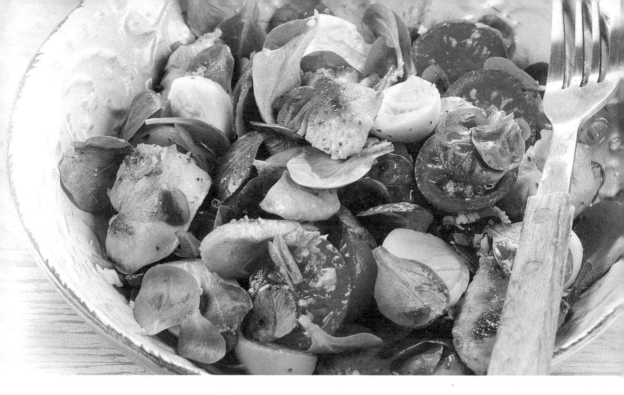

Chicken Lunch Salad

If you have any type of cooked chicken on hand, it can be used instead of the grilled breast listed in the ingredients. Assemble your lunch plate and you are good to go.

Ingredients

- 2 C baby spinach leaves
- 2 Grilled Chicken Breasts, cut into bite-sized pieces
- ½ C cherry tomatoes, cut in half
- 2 green onions, sliced thinly
- 2 Perfectly Hard Boiled Eggs, cut into quarters
- 2 T vinaigrette (or other keto dressing of choice
- ½ C Fermented Cauliflower

Preparation

1. Divide spinach, chicken, tomatoes, green onions and boiled egg between 4 salad bowls.

2. Drizzle vinaigrette or dressing of choice over-top and place fermented cauliflower pieces on the side of each bowl.

Yield: 4 Servings

Nutritional Information:

- Calories/serving: 165
- Net carbs: 2g
- Total Carbs: 4g
- Total Fat: 9g
- Fiber: 2g
- Protein: 16g

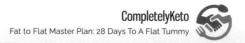

CompletelyKeto
Fat to Flat Master Plan: 28 Days To A Flat Tummy

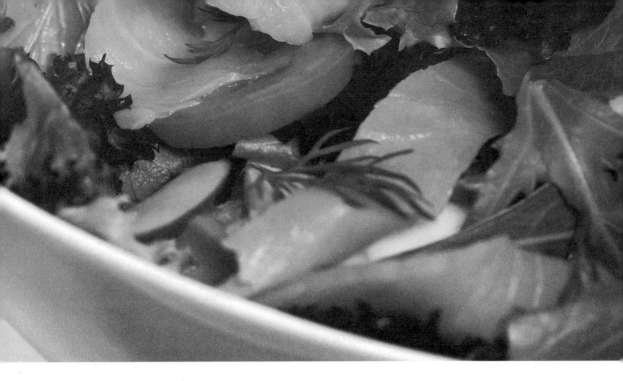

Smoked Salmon Salad

Ingredients

- 6 C mixed greens
- 1 C cherry tomatoes, halved
- 2 green onions (scallions), thinly sliced
- ¼ C snipped fresh herbs, optional
- 3 T freshly squeezed lemon juice
- ¼ C extra-virgin olive oil
- 12 oz smoked salmon, thinly sliced

Preparation

1. Divide mixed greens, cherry tomatoes. Sliced green onion and snipped herbs (if using) between 4 salad bowls.

2. Whisk lemon juice and olive oil. Divide the salmon into 4 portions and tuck the thin slices in amongst the greens in each bowl.

3. Drizzle the lemon dressing over each of the salads. Serve with one or two Fermented Dill Pickles on the side and enjoy!

Yield: 4 Servings

Nutritional Information:

- Calories/serving: 432
- Net carbs: 6g
- Total Carbs: 7g
- Total Fat: 32g
- Fiber: 1g
- Protein: 26g

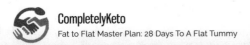

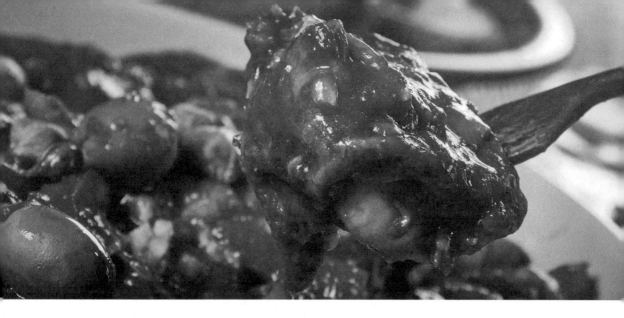

Haddock with Olives, Capers and Tomatoes

You can throw this dish together and get it into the oven in five minutes for an easy lunch. Bake for another 20 and you will be sitting down to a nourishing, hot meal in the middle of the day!

Ingredients

- 1 ½ lb haddock fillets, cut in half
- Grinding of pink Himalayan salt and black peppercorns
- 20 green olives, pitted
- 2 T capers
- 1 ½ C canned crushed tomatoes
- ½ C fish broth (or vegetable broth)
- A few drops of liquid stevia

Preparation

1. Pre-heat oven to 350 F.
2. Place fillets in baking dish and season with salt and pepper. Distribute capers and olives evenly over-top. Mix crushed tomatoes, broth with stevia. Pour over-top making sure the ingredients in the baking dish are covered with the tomato mixture.
3. Place dish on the middle rack of the pre-heated oven and braise in the oven for 20 minutes. The internal temperature of the fish should reach 145 F when done. Serve and enjoy for lunch or dinner.

Yield: 4 Servings

Nutritional Information:

- Calories/serving: 198
- Total Carbs: 8g
- Fiber: 3g
- Net carbs: 5g
- Total Fat: 4g
- Protein: 34g

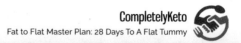

CompletelyKeto

Fat to Flat Master Plan: 28 Days To A Flat Tummy

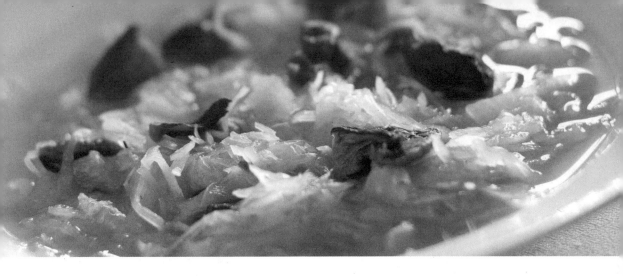

Sauerkraut Chicken Soup

Traditional Russian Sauerkraut Soup would include potato but here, we leave it out of the ingredients list. The flavor is still superb in this keto version of a Russian classic!

Ingredients

- 2 T extra virgin olive oil
- 1 yellow cooking onion, medium dice
- 6 C chicken broth
- 2 C Fermented Sauerkraut
- 1 C shredded cabbage
- ¼ C fresh dill leaves (or 1 T dried dill)
- 1 C cooked chicken, cut into bite-sized chunks or shredded
- 1 C mushrooms
- 4 T full fat Greek yogurt, for garnish

Preparation

1. Heat 1 T of the oil in a heavy bottomed soup pot. Sauté onion until soft and translucent. Add broth, sauerkraut, shredded cabbage and dill. Raise the heat under the pot and simmer until the cabbage is cooked.

2. Meanwhile, sauté the sliced mushrooms until cooked. Set aside.

3. Add cooked chicken to the soup pot and simmer for a few minutes more until everything is heated through. Ladle into 4 bowls. Divide the cooked mushrooms between the bowls, garnish with the Greek yogurt, serve and enjoy!

Yield: 4 Servings

Nutritional Information:

- Calories/serving: 232
- Total Carbs: 8g
- Fiber: 3g
- Net carbs: 5g
- Total Fat: 15g
- Protein: 10g

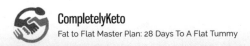

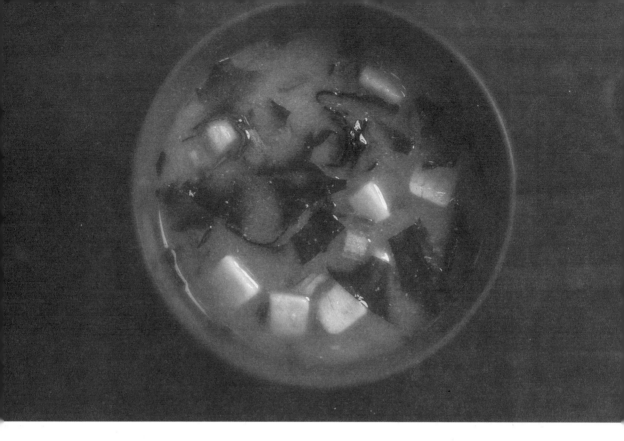

Miso Soup

Ingredients

- 1 sheet nori, cut into smaller pieces
- 3 T white or yellow miso paste
- ½ C green chard, roughly chopped
- 3 green onions, thinly sliced
- ½ C firm tofu, cut into small cubes

Preparation

1. Place miso into a small bowl and add a small amount of hot water. Whisk until the miso is dissolved and the mixture is smooth in texture. Set aside.

2. Pour broth into a saucepan and bring to a simmer.

3. Add chard, green onion and tofu. Simmer for 5 minutes.

4. Add nori and stir. Remove from heat and stir in the miso mixture. Serve while hot.

Yield: 2 Servings

Nutritional Information:

- Calories/serving: 120
- Total Carbs: 13g
- Fiber: 5g
- Net carbs: 8g
- Total Fat: 4g
- Protein: 11g

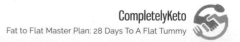

CompletelyKeto

Fat to Flat Master Plan: 28 Days To A Flat Tummy

Hot and Sour Soup

Ingredients

- 1 T extra virgin olive oil
- 1 C sliced cremini mushrooms
- 2 green onions (thinly sliced), reserve 1 T for garnish
- 1½ T fresh ginger root, grated or minced
- 2 garlic cloves, minced or pushed through a press
- 8 C chicken or veggie broth
- ½ tsp red pepper flakes
- ¼ C unseasoned rice vinegar
- ¼ C gluten free tamari sauce
- 4 eggs, lightly beaten
- Grinding of pink Himalayan salt and black peppercorns, to taste

Preparation

1. Add oil to a large heavy bottomed pot over a medium-high heat. Add the mushrooms, scallions, ginger and garlic. Cook and stir for 1-2 minutes to infuse the flavor.

2. Add the broth, red pepper flakes, vinegar and tamari sauce. Bring to a boil, then reduce the heat and allow to simmer for about 10 minutes or until the mushrooms are tender.

3. Stir the soup in a circular motion in one direction, then drizzle in the eggs in a thin and steady stream while continue stirring. This will cause the beaten egg to form ribbons in the hot soup.

4. Ladle the soup into bowls and garnish each bowl the remaining green onion slices.

Yield: 8 Servings

Nutritional Information:

- Calories/serving: 113
- Total Carbs: 2g
- Fiber: 1g
- Net carbs: 1g
- Total Fat: 4g
- Protein: 5g

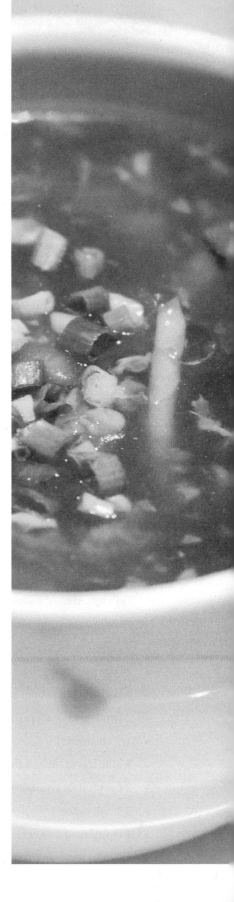

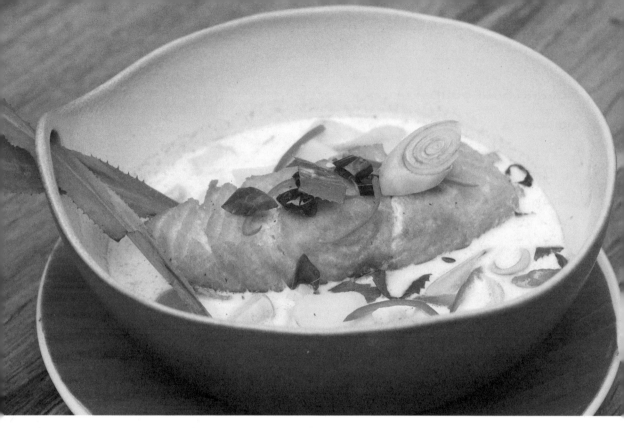

Tom Kha (Coconut/Salmon Soup)

This coconut/salmon soup is very filling and full of flavor. You can cut the salmon into cubes or serve one larger piece in each bowl. If you like heat, then add an extra pepper (or 2)! If less heat is desired, remove and discard the seeds.

Ingredients

- 1 ½ lb salmon fillet, skinless
- ½ tsp pink Himalayan salt flakes
- ½ lb mixed mushrooms (oyster, shiitake, Portobello, etc.)
- ½ yellow cooking onion, small dice
- 3 garlic cloves, minced or pushed through a press
- 3" piece of fresh ginger root, peeled and minced
- 1 hot red chili pepper more if you like heat, sliced lengthwise with seeds included
- 2 lemongrass stalks
- 1 T coconut oil
- 8 lime leaves (or zest from 2 limes)
- 2 cans full fat coconut milk
- 2 T fish sauce
- 1 tsp allowed sweetener (or a few drops liquid stevia)
- Cilantro leaves for garnish, if desired

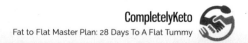

CompletelyKeto
Fat to Flat Master Plan: 28 Days To A Flat Tummy

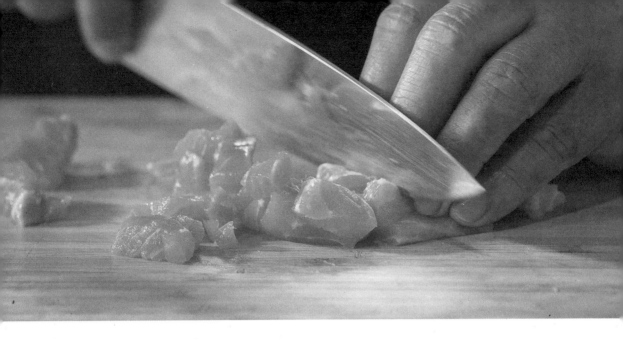

Preparation

1. Slice mushrooms and/or tear the clusters (like shiitake mushroom clusters) into smaller chunks.

2. Cut salmon into 1" cubes (or 6 larger pieces as pictured), place in a bowl and sprinkle ½ tsp of the salt over-top.

3. Trim the outer part of the lemongrass stalks away. The top 2/3 of each stalk will be a bit tougher so cut this part off and discard. Slice the remaining soft yellow lemongrass into thin rings.

4. Melt the coconut oil in a heavy bottomed saucepan over medium high heat and sauté the diced onion for two minutes then add the garlic and ginger and continue to sauté for another 3 minutes or until everything has softened.

5. Add the pepper, lemongrass, lime leaves (or zest) and pour in the coconut milk. Stir in the fish sauce and sweetener.

6. Bring the liquid to the boil then adjust the heat so it's just simmering. Allow the soup to simmer for 8 minutes the increase the heat.

7. Add the salmon and mushrooms to the pot and when the liquid comes to the boil, once again reduce the heat so the liquid is just simmering. Allow the soup to simmer until the salmon is cooked through and just beginning to get flaky. This won't take long so keep a close eye on the soup as the salmon can be easily overcooked.

8. Squeeze the juice from one lime and add the juice to the soup. Taste and correct the seasoning, if necessary. Serve the soup garnished with chopped cilantro leaves, if desired.

Yield: 6 Servings

Nutritional Information:

- Total Calories/Serving: 238
- Total Carbs: 6g
- Fiber: 2g
- Net Carbs: 4g
- Total Fat: 12g
- Protein: 25g

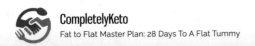

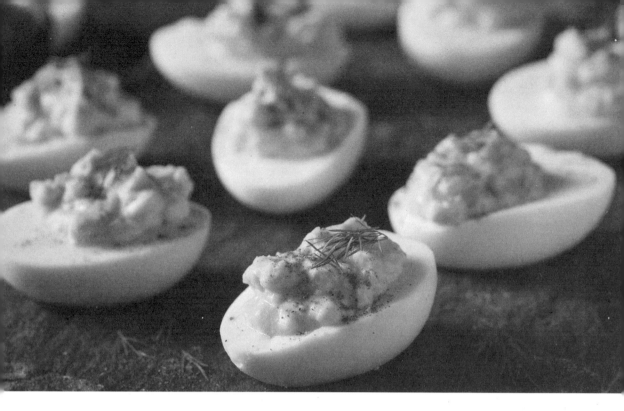

Deviled Dilly Eggs

I usually make a larger batch when making devilled eggs. They are popular lunch time fare in my house and disappear quickly!

Ingredients

- 12 Perfectly hard Boiled Eggs, cut in half lengthwise
- 6 T full fat mayonnaise
- 2 tsp Dijon mustard
- 1 T dried dill
- Grinding of pink Himalayan salt and black peppercorns, to taste
- Garnish with a sprinkle of paprika and dill, if desired

Preparation

1. Remove yolks and mix with mayo, mustard, dill, salt and pepper.
2. Fill the egg white cavities with the yolk mixture and garnish with a light sprinkle of paprika and dill, if desired.

Yield: 12 Servings

Nutritional Information:

- Calories/serving: 124
- Net carbs: 1g
- Total Carbs: 1g
- Total Fat: 12g
- Fiber: 0g
- Protein: 6g

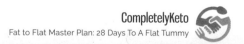

CompletelyKeto
Fat to Flat Master Plan: 28 Days To A Flat Tummy

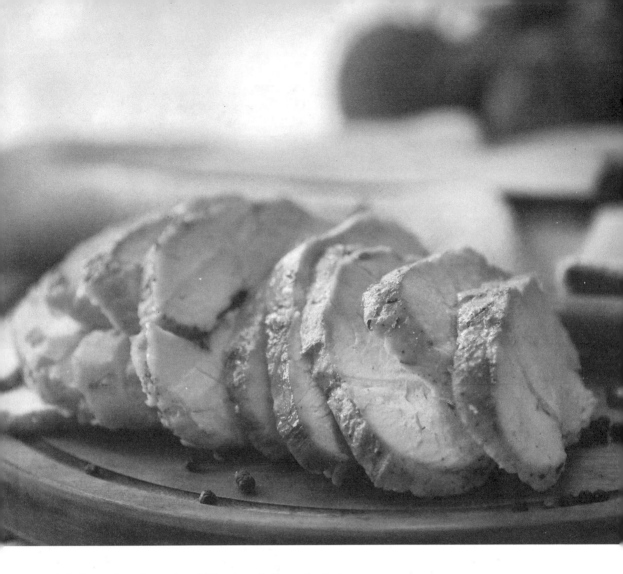

Chicken (or Smoked Turkey) Sandwich

Ingredients

- 2 Keto Cloud Bread
- 1 T Keto Mayonnaise (full fat and no sugar)
- 2 oz. smoked chicken slices or smoked turkey slices (from the deli)

Preparation

1. Assemble sandwich and enjoy!

Yield: 1 Serving

Nutritional Information:

- Total Calories/serving: 316 *(with Keto Cloud Bread)*
- Total Carbs: 3g
- Fiber: 0g
- Net Carbs: 3g
- Total Fat: 23g
- Protein: 20g

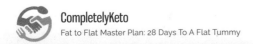

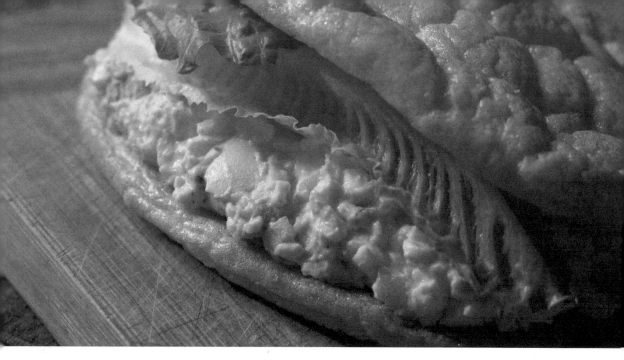

Egg Salad Sandwich

I love a bit of curry in my egg salad but skip this spice if it's not on your list of favorites.

Ingredients

- 2 Keto Cloud Bread pieces
- 1 Perfectly Hard Boiled Egg
- 1 T approved mayonnaise
- ¼ tsp Dijon mustard
- 1 green onion (scallion), thinly sliced or 2 T red onion, minced
- ½ tsp curry powder
- 1 Romaine lettuce leaf, (or a few mixed greens)
- Himalayan salt and black pepper (to taste)

Preparation

1. Mash hardboiled egg with a fork and mix in the mayonnaise, Dijon mustard, green onion and curry powder. Correct the seasoning with salt and pepper.

2. Spread the egg mixture on one piece of cloud bread. Top with the Romaine lettuce and cover with the second piece of Cloud Bread. Cut in half and serve.

Yield: Serves 1

Nutritional Information:

- Total Calories/serving: 245
- Total Carbs: 6 g
- Fiber: 5 g
- Total Fat: 20 g
- Protein: 10 g

CompletelyKeto
Fat to Flat Master Plan: 28 Days To A Flat Tummy

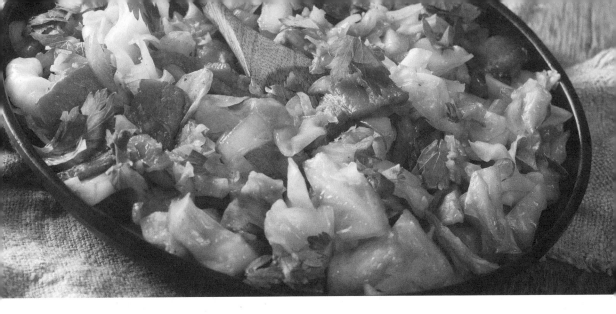

Sauerkraut, Cabbage and Turkey Bacon Stir-fry

This simple stir-fry makes a quick lunch on its own or a perfect side-dish at dinner time. We like the added tang of sauerkraut in this easy to prepare recipe.

Ingredients

- 1 T plus ½ T extra-virgin olive oil
- ¼ C cooking onion, small dice
- 2 C cabbage, shredded
- 2 C sauerkraut
- 4 strips thick-cut turkey bacon
- 4 eggs

Preparation

1. Heat oil in a wok or heavy bottomed skillet over medium high heat. Add diced onion and stir-fry for a few minutes until the onion is softened and translucent.

2. Add the cabbage and stir-fry for 4 or 5 minutes until the cabbage is wilted and cooked. Add the sauerkraut and stir-fry until everything is heated through. Toss in the prepared bacon and stir-fry for one more minute. Remove from heat and keep warm.

3. Heat remaining oil in a heavy bottomed skillet. Fry eggs to your liking.

4. Divide cabbage/sauerkraut mixture between 4 bowls and top each with a fried egg. Serve immediately.

Yield: 4 Servings

Nutritional Information:

- Calories/serving: 197
- Total Carbs: 8g
- Fiber: 1g
- Net carbs: 7g
- Total Fat: 13g
- Protein: 13g

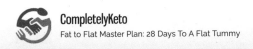

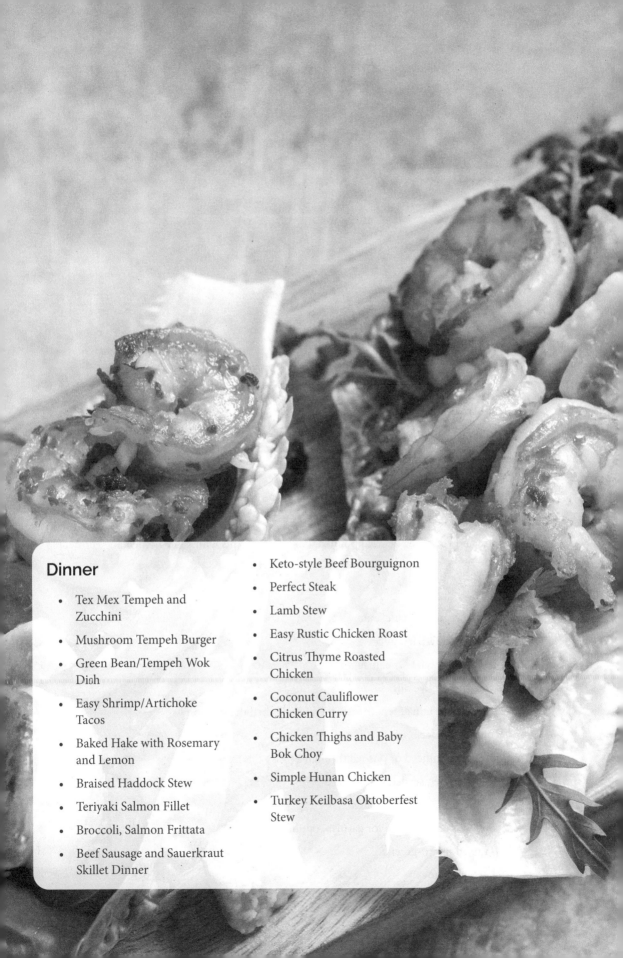

Dinner

- Tex Mex Tempeh and Zucchini
- Mushroom Tempeh Burger
- Green Bean/Tempeh Wok Dish
- Easy Shrimp/Artichoke Tacos
- Baked Hake with Rosemary and Lemon
- Braised Haddock Stew
- Teriyaki Salmon Fillet
- Broccoli, Salmon Frittata
- Beef Sausage and Sauerkraut Skillet Dinner

- Keto-style Beef Bourguignon
- Perfect Steak
- Lamb Stew
- Easy Rustic Chicken Roast
- Citrus Thyme Roasted Chicken
- Coconut Cauliflower Chicken Curry
- Chicken Thighs and Baby Bok Choy
- Simple Hunan Chicken
- Turkey Keilbasa Oktoberfest Stew

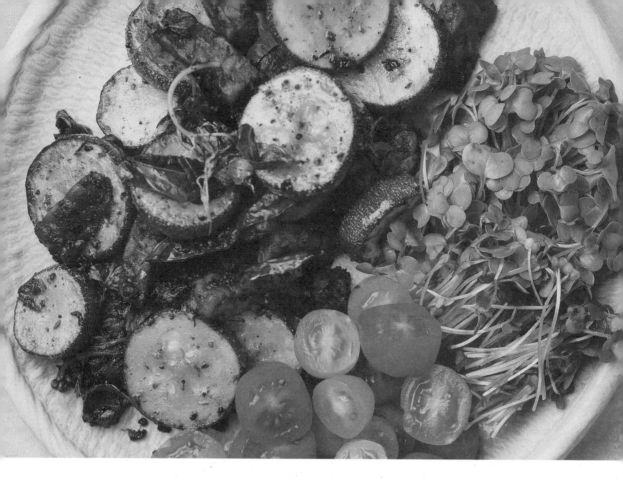

Tex Mex Tempeh and Zucchini

Here's a Tex Mex combo you thought you'd never see; tempeh and zucchini. But give it a try with an open mind and you won't be disappointed. I like to serve this with some homemade Fermented Red Salsa on the side.

Ingredients

- ¾ C broth (vegetable, chicken or beef)
- 2 T gluten-free Tamari sauce
- ¼ C freshly squeezed lime juice
- 2 T extra virgin olive oil
- 8 oz tempeh, cut in half lengthwise, then into ½ inch thick strips
- 2 tsp onion powder
- 2 garlic cloves, minced or pushed through a press
- 1 jalapeño pepper, seeded and minced
- 2 small zucchini, cut into rounds
- 2 T chopped fresh cilantro for garnish, optional
- 1 ½ C mixed micro-greens
- 1 C cherry tomatoes

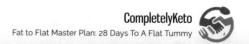
CompletelyKeto
Fat to Flat Master Plan: 28 Days To A Flat Tummy

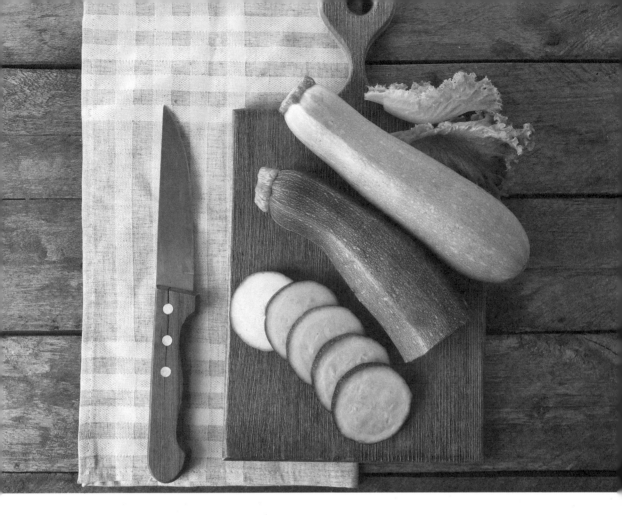

Preparation

1. Mix tamari. Lime juice and broth together. Set a heavy bottomed skillet or wok skillet over medium high heat and add about half of the oil, ¼ C of the broth mixture and the tempeh strips. Stir-fry occasionally until the tempeh is starting to brown on most sides.

2. The broth will be soaked up as you stir-fry. This process will take about 10 minutes. You will need to stir-fry more often as the liquid lessens in the wok.

3. Pour in a bit more of the stock mixture if needed to keep the skillet moist. Remove the browned tempeh and set aside (keep warm).

4. Pour the remaining oil into the pan. Add the garlic, jalapeño pepper and onion powder. Stir-fry for two minutes. Add the zucchini and tempeh and stir-fry about one minute.

5. Divide into 4 servings, garnish with cilantro if desired, plate and serve with mixed greens and cherry tomatoes.

Yield: 4 Servings

Nutritional Information:

- Calories/serving: 207
- Net carbs: 10g
- Total Carbs: 12g
- Total Fat: 13g
- Fiber: 2g
- Protein: 15g

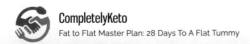

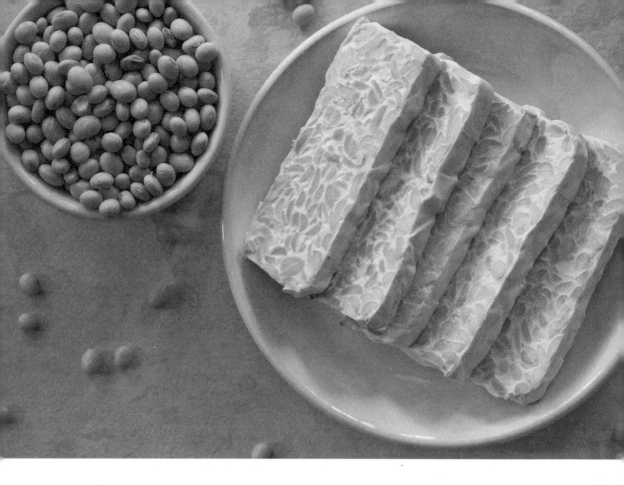

Mushroom Tempeh Burger

I've included instructions for stove-top cooking, but you could easily fire up the BBQ to grill the tempeh and Portobello mushrooms. Either way you will end up with a flavorful and juicy vegan burger tonight!

Ingredients

- 6 oz tempeh
- ¼ C broth (vegetable, chicken or beef)
- T gluten free tamari sauce, no sugar
- 1 ½ T freshly squeezed lemon (or lime) juice
- ½ tsp garlic powder (or granules)
- 1 tsp onion powder
- ½ tsp dried thyme
- 2 T extra virgin olive oil
- 4 whole Portobello mushrooms, cleaned and stem removed
- 1 medium tomato
- 2 large flat leaf lettuce leaves
- Fermented Hot Sauce, optional

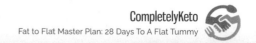

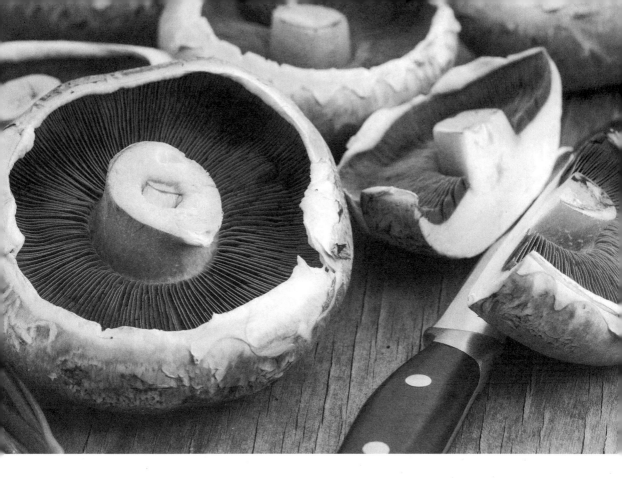

Preparation

1. Cut 2, ½" thick slices (horizontally) from a block of tempeh; each slice should weigh approximately 3 oz.

2. Place tempeh slices in a wide mouth bowl.

3. Whisk broth, tamari, lemon juice, garlic powder, onion powder and thyme. Pour over tempeh and refrigerate for at least one hour.

4. Brush both sides of the prepared Portobello mushrooms using 1 T of the olive oil. Heat heavy bottomed skillet over medium high heat and fry the mushrooms for 2 or 3 minutes on each side until done. Remove from heat and keep warm.

5. Remove tempeh from marinade. Heat remaining olive oil in the hot skillet over medium high heat. Fry tempeh slices for 2 or 3 minutes on each side.

6. Assemble a burger by layering a slice of tempeh, a tomato slice and a leaf of lettuce between 2 of the cooked Portobello mushrooms. Drizzle a bit of Fermented Hot Sauce overtop the tempeh when layering the ingredients, if desired. Repeat process to make the second burger.

Yield: 2 Servings

Nutritional Information:

- Calories/serving: 385
- Total Carbs: 18g
- Fiber: 6g
- Net carbs: 12g
- Total Fat: 25g
- Protein: 24g

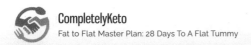

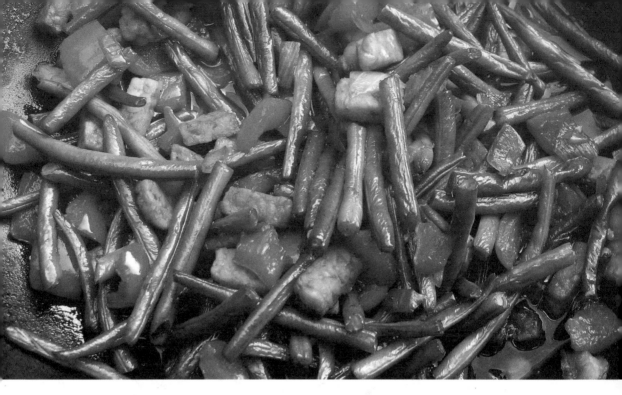

Green Bean/Tempeh Wok Dish

Tempeh provides a fermented food that is full of flavor and supports a healthy gut. Give it a try; I think you will like it! You can use my Keto Teriyaki Sauce for this dish or purchase a commercially available alternative that is made with no sugar. Serve over Cauliflower rice and enjoy.

Ingredients

- 1 T extra-virgin olive oil
- 1 C green beans, cut into 2 " pieces
- 1 red bell pepper, medium dice
- 12 oz tempeh, cut into bite-sized cubes
- ¼ C Keto Teriyaki Sauce

Preparation

1. Heat oil in a heavy bottomed skillet or Wok.
2. Add green beans and stir-fry until beans are cooked but still a nice bright green in color and remain a bit crunchy. When almost done add the red pepper and tempeh.
3. Continue to stir-fry for another few minutes until everything is heated through.

Yield: 4 Servings

Nutritional Information:

- Calories/serving: 237
- Net carbs: 10g
- Total Carbs: 13g
- Total Fat: 13g
- Fiber: 3g
- Protein: 20g

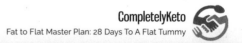
CompletelyKeto
Fat to Flat Master Plan: 28 Days To A Flat Tummy

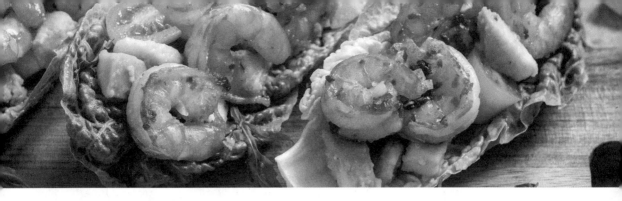

Easy Shrimp/Artichoke Tacos

When an easy lunch or quick dinner is required here's the perfect recipe. I keep frozen shrimp and canned artichokes on hand for just such an emergency!

Ingredients

- 16 large shrimp, peeled and deveined
- 1 tsp chili powder
- 1 tsp smoked paprika
- ½ tsp cumin powder
- 2 T extra virgin olive oil
- 2 garlic cloves, minced or pushed through a press
- Grinding of pink Himalayan salt and black peppercorns, to taste
- 1 C canned artichoke hearts, cut into bite-sized chunks
- ½ C heirloom cherry tomatoes, cut into chunks
- 12 romaine lettuce leaves
- Juice from ½ lemon (about 2 T)

Preparation

1. Place prepared shrimp in a bowl. Sprinkle spices over-top and toss shrimp until they are evenly coated with the spices.
2. Heat oil in a heavy bottomed skillet or wok over medium high heat. Add the shrimp and minced garlic when the oil is hot. Stir-fry the shrimp until they are curled up and pink. They will cook quickly so be careful not to overdo them as they will become rubbery.
3. Place 3 Romaine leaves on each of 4 plates.
4. Divide the artichoke chunks and chopped cherry tomatoes evenly, between all of the lettuce leaves. Place 4 shrimp in each leaf and squeeze the half lemon, briefly, over-top each taco.

Yield: 4 Servings

Nutritional Information:

- Calories/serving: 157
- Total Carbs: 9g
- Fiber: 4g
- Net carbs: 5g
- Total Fat: 8g
- Protein: 42g

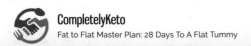

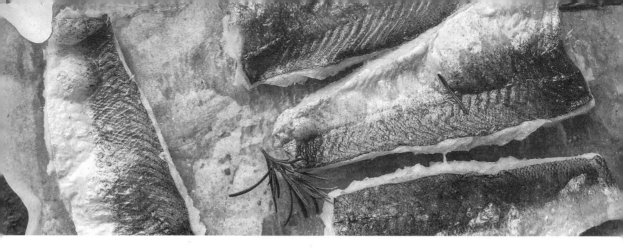

Baked Hake with Rosemary, Lemon and Capers

I've selected hake for this recipe because it's readily available where I shop but you could easily substitute any white fleshed fish.

Ingredients

- 2 cloves garlic, minced or pushed through a press
- 2 sprigs rosemary, leaves removed and minced
- ¼ C capers
- 1 teaspoon lemon zest
- 2 T extra-virgin olive oil
- 2 lb (4 pieces) hake fillets
- Grinding of pink Himalayan salt and black peppercorns, to taste

Preparation

1. Make a marinade by mixing the garlic, rosemary, capers, lemon zest, and olive oil in a bowl. Roll the fish in the mixture. Marinate in the fridge for 10-15 minutes.

2. Preheat oven to 375 degrees.

3. Line a rimmed baking sheet with foil and place the fish in the pan, allowing the marinade to cling to fish surface as much as possible. Cover with the remaining marinade. Season with salt and pepper. Drizzle juice from lemon over-top the fish.

4. Bake on the middle rack of the pre-heated oven for 15 minutes or until the internal temperature of the fish reaches 145F.

5. Allow fish to rest for a few minutes then transfer to 4 plates and serve with veggies on the side.

Yield: 4 Servings

Nutritional Information:

- Calories/serving: 248
- Net carbs: 1g
- Total Carbs: 1g
- Total Fat: 9g
- Fiber: 0g
- Protein: 40g

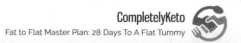

CompletelyKeto

Fat to Flat Master Plan: 28 Days To A Flat Tummy

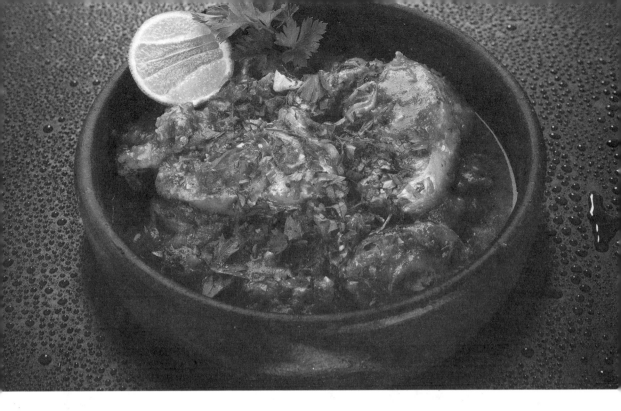

Braised Haddock Stew

This fish stew is full of flavor with a tomato/coconut milk broth that pairs well with the light taste of red haddock. A drizzle of fresh lime juice before it goes to the table brightens the flavor of this lightly curried casserole. I like to ladle this stew over Cauliflower "Rice"

Ingredients

- 4 Haddock fillets (about 1 lb)
- Fresh juice from 1 lime (about 2T)
- 2 T extra virgin olive oil
- Grinding of pink Himalayan salt and black peppercorns
- ½ yellow cooking onion, small dice
- 1 red bell pepper, seeded and sliced thinly
- 2 garlic cloves, minced or pushed through a press
- ½ tsp ground cumin
- 1 T paprika salt
- ½ tsp cayenne, less if you don't want heat or more if you do
- 1 tsp pink Himalayan
- 1 C crushed (canned) tomatoes
- 1 C full fat coconut milk
- 2 T fresh lime juice
- ¼ C chopped fresh cilantro leaves

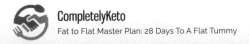

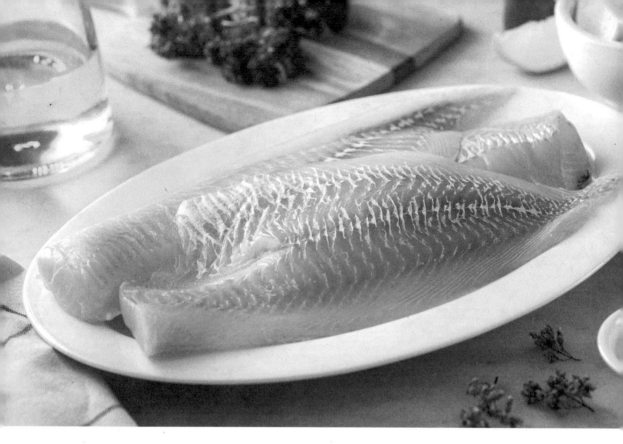

Preparation

1. Place haddock in a bowl. Make a marinade by whisking olive oil, lime juice salt and pepper. Pour over the fish and refrigerate for 20 minutes.

2. Remove fillets from marinade and pat dry. Heat the olive oil in a large heavy bottomed skillet over medium high heat. Sauté the fish for 3 minutes on one side and flip. Sauté for another 3 or 4 minutes or until the internal temperature reaches 145 F. Remove fish and keep warm.

3. Add 1 T of olive oil to the same skillet and sauté the onions for 4 minutes until they begin to soften. Add the red bell pepper and sauté for 3 minutes more.

4. Add the garlic, cumin, paprika, salt and cayenne. Continue to sauté for 4 minutes more.

5. Pour in the crushed tomatoes, full fat coconut milk and fish broth. Stir while the liquid comes up to the boil. Re-adjust the heat so the broth is just simmering. Simmer for 15 minutes.

6. Return the cooked fish to the skillet and re-heat for a few minutes. Squeeze fresh lime juice over-top and ladle the stew into six wide bowls. Garnish with cilantro leaves and serve.

Yield: 6 Servings

Nutritional Information:

- Total Calories/Serving: 254
- Total Carbs: 11g
- Fiber: 3g
- Net Carbs: 8g
- Total Fat: 14g
- Protein: 21g

CompletelyKeto
Fat to Flat Master Plan: 28 Days To A Flat Tummy

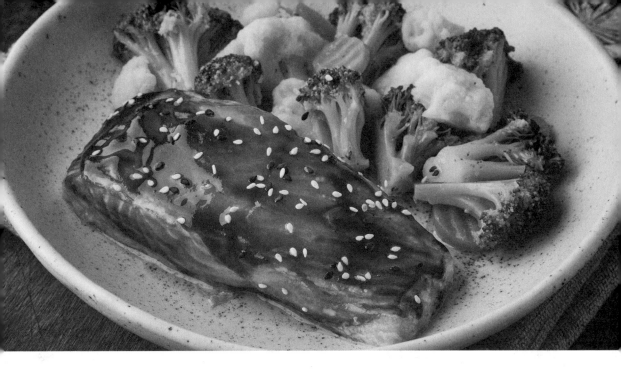

Teriyaki Salmon Fillet

Dinner or lunch is done quickly when salmon fillets are on the menu. If you already have my home-made Keto Teriyaki Sauce on hand then prep will be even faster!

Ingredients

- 1 lb salmon fillets
- ¼ C Keto Teriyaki Sauce
- 2 C cauliflower and broccoli florets

Preparation

1. Pre-heat oven to 350F.
2. Place salmon fillets close together, on a piece of aluminum foil. Pour teriyaki sauce over-top. Fold the foil to make a sealed packet around the fillets. Put the packet on a rimmed baking sheet and place the sheet on the middle rack of the pre-heated oven. Bake for 20 minutes. The internal temperature of the fillets should reach 145F.
3. While the salmon is baking, prepare the cauliflower and broccoli florets. Steam them over boiling water until they are cooked but still firm in texture.
4. This takes only a matter of minutes so you can allow the salmon to rest while you cook the veggies. Divide the salmon and florets amongst 4 plates and serve immediately.

Yield: 4 Servings

Nutritional Information:

- Total Calories/Serving: 321
- Total Carbs: 6g
- Fiber: 2g
- Net Carbs: 4g
- Total Fat: 15g
- Protein: 41g

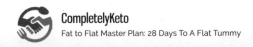

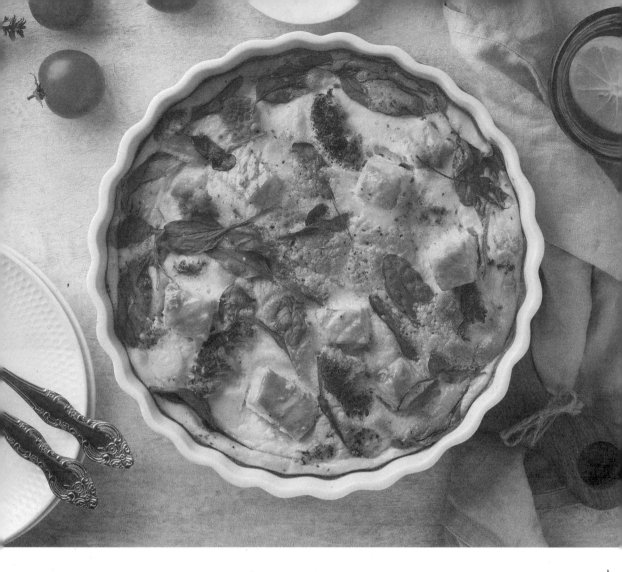

Broccoli, Spinach and Salmon Frittata

I've used fresh salmon fillets in this frittata, but you can easily substitute sugar free smoked salmon and skip the time it takes to bake the fillets.

Ingredients

- 2 salmon fillets (about ½ lb)
- 1 T lemon juice
- Grinding of pink Himalayan salt and black peppercorns
- 6 eggs, whisked
- ½ C full fat canned coconut milk
- 1 tsp onion powder
- 1 C broccoli florets
- 1 C baby spinach leaves
- 1 T fresh herbs of choice, optional

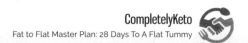

CompletelyKeto
Fat to Flat Master Plan: 28 Days To A Flat Tummy

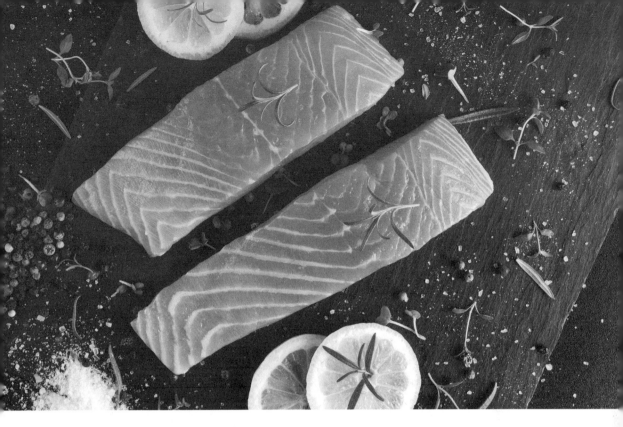

Preparation

1. Preheat oven to 350F

2. Season salmon with salt and pepper. Place on parchment lined, rimmed baking sheet and place on the middle rack of the pre-heated oven. Bake for 20 minutes. Cool and cut salmon into bite sized cubes. Set aside. Leave the oven on.

3. While the salmon is in the oven, steam the broccoli for a few minutes until it is tender but still is a nice green color and has a bit of crunch. Brush a pie plate lightly with oil. Arrange broccoli evenly around pie plate. Do the same with the baby spinach.

4. Add onion powder and coconut cream to whisked egg, whisking well. Season with a grinding of salt and pepper.

5. Carefully pour the egg mixture into the pie plate around the broccoli and spinach. Spread cubed salmon evenly around the frittata, allowing it to rest into the egg mixture.

6. Place the frittata on the middle rack of the oven and bake for 20 minutes or until the egg is set.

7. Allow to rest for a few minutes before cutting into wedges. Garnish with fresh lemon juice and herbs, if desired. Serve immediately.

Yield: 4 Servings

Nutritional Information:

- Calories/serving: 264
- Net carbs: 5g
- Total Carbs: 6g
- Total Fat: 18g
- Fiber: 1g
- Protein: 16g

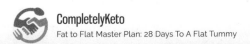

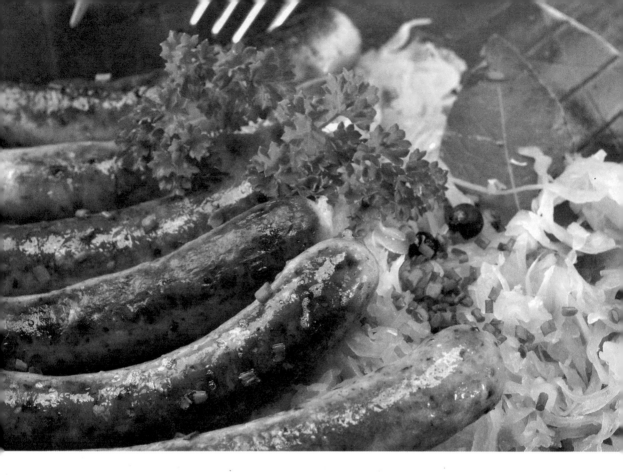

Beef Sausage and Sauerkraut Skillet Dinner

Great for breakfast, lunch or dinner, this meal tastes great and requires no fussing at all!

Ingredients

- 8 beef sausages (3 oz each)
- 2 C Keto Sauerkraut

Preparation

1. Fry sausages in a stick-free, heavy bottomed skillet over medium high heat. Roll them around occasionally so all sides get nicely browned and the sausages cook evenly.

2. The internal temperature should read 165 F when the sausages are done. Remove from the skillet and keep warm.

3. Return skillet to the heat and add the sauerkraut. Stir while kraut heats up. Divide sauerkraut and sausages between 4 plates and serve.

Yield: 4 Servings

Nutritional Information:

- Calories/serving: 393
- Net carbs: 8g
- Total Carbs: 9g
- Total Fat: 42g
- Fiber: 1g
- Protein: 28g

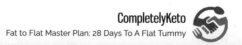
CompletelyKeto
Fat to Flat Master Plan: 28 Days To A Flat Tummy

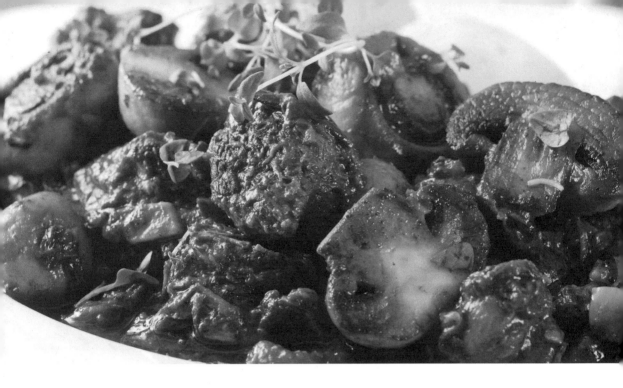

Keto-style Beef Bourguignon

This Fat to Flat Masterplan version of beef bourguignon is outstanding when served over Cauliflower Mash. This traditional beef stew is super yummy!

Since beef is limited on this program, I want you to enjoy every bite when it shows up in the menu plan. Here's one of my favorite beef meals ... enjoy!

Ingredients

- 4 thick-cut, turkey bacon slices, diced
- 1 ½ lb beef stew meat, cut into I" cubes
- 1 T extra-virgin olive oil, divided in 1/2T
- ½ medium yellow cooking onion, medium dice
- 1 celery stock, small dice
- 2 garlic cloves, minced or pushed through a press
- ½ tsp xanthan gum
- 2 C beef broth
- 2 T tomato paste
- ½ tsp dried thyme leaves
- 1 bay leaf
- ½ tsp pink Himalayan salt flakes
- ½ tsp ground black peppercorns
- 1 C mushrooms (white or cremini), cut in half
- 1 T fresh chopped parsley, for garnish if desired

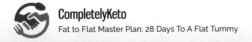

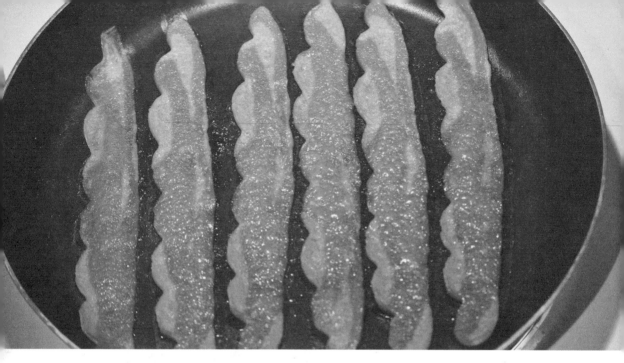

Preparation

1. Pre-heat oven to 325 F.

2. Heat a large enameled cast iron dutch oven over medium high heat. Add turkey bacon and fry until crisp. Remove bacon leaving the rendered fat behind. Drain the strips on paper towel.

3. Add beef and brown on all sides (do this in two batches so beef cubes aren't crowded (they shouldn't touch each other). Remove and keep warm.

4. Add ½ T oil to the pot and sauté onion and celery until they soften and the onion becomes translucent. Stir in the garlic.

5. Whisk tomato paste, thyme, salt, pepper, beef broth and xanthan gum. Pour into pot and simmer until the sauce thickens slightly. Add the bacon and browned beef back into the pot along with the bay leaf. Give everything a stir then place the covered pot onto the middle rack of the pre-heated oven and bake for one hour. Stir, uncover the pot and bake for another hour or until the meat is very tender. You could also cook in a slow cooker (crock-pot) on low for 6-8 hours.

6. Just before you are ready to serve the meal, melt the remaining ½ T of extra-virgin olive oil over medium high heat in a large, heavy bottomed skillet. Sauté the mushroom until cooked and nicely browned. Stir the mushrooms into the stew.

7. Remove bay leaf and ladle the beef bourguignon over-top Cauliflower Mash. Garnish with parsley (if desired) and serve.

Yield: 4 Servings

Nutritional Information:

- Total Calories/serving: 294
- Total Carbs: 6g
- Fiber: 2g
- Net Carbs: 4g
- Total Fat: 11g
- Protein: 42g

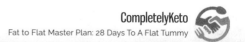
CompletelyKeto
Fat to Flat Master Plan: 28 Days To A Flat Tummy

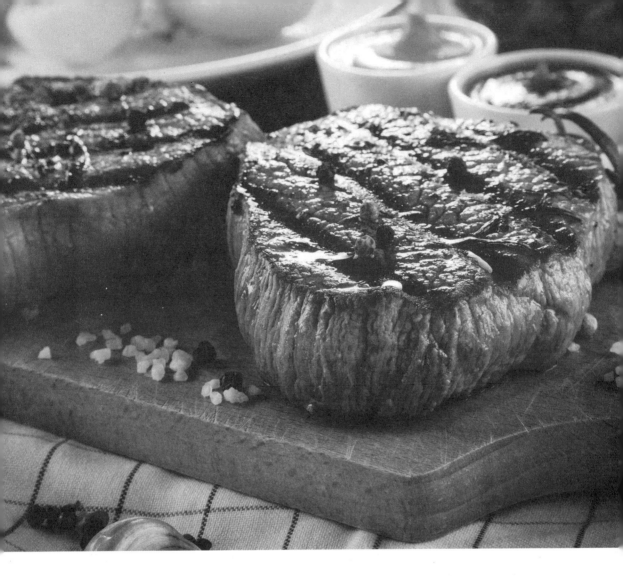

Perfect Steak

Beef is an allowed food on the Fat to Flat Masterplan program; however, the emphasis is on fermented foods in combination with fish, fowl, tofu, tempeh and eggs when it comes to daily protein intake. I've purposely limited beef, so when it does show up in the menu plan, I want you to really enjoy your meal. So… what could be better than perfectly cooked steak!

Fire up the BBQ, indoor grill or just get out a heavy cast iron grill pan (the kind with ridges). While I really enjoy the added flavor from using the BBQ to cook steak, I also have no problem with the stove-top method using a grill pan.

You can still get some of that yummy charring indoors. However you choose to cook your steak, be sure to choose a nicely marbled piece of meat, that's at least one inch thick (preferably 1.5"). My favorite cuts include: beef tenderloin, T-bone, porterhouse, strip loin, rib-eye and prime rib.

Ingredients

- 4, 4-6 oz steaks
- Grinding of pink Himalayan salt and black peppercorns

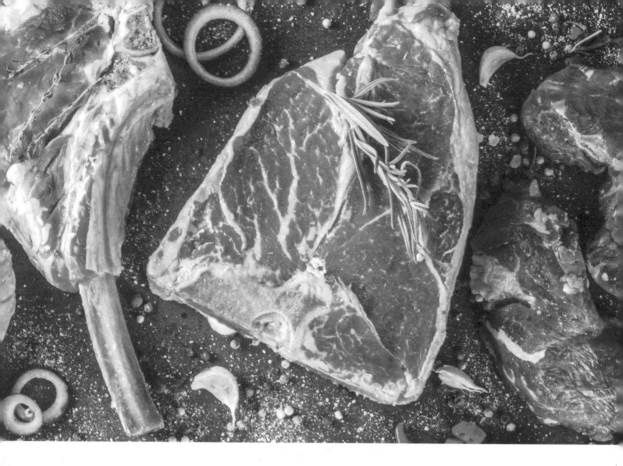

Preparation

1. BBQ Method: Pre-heat the grill to high and the sear the steaks for 2 minutes on each side with the lid open. Then lower the heat to medium, close the lid and continue grilling for 2 or 3 more minutes per side.

2. The time will vary depending on the thickness of the steaks and your preference for "doneness". You will want to remove the steaks from the grill when the internal temperature reaches 120 F in the center for rare or ... 130 F for medium-rare. Let the steaks rest for a few minutes during which time the internal temp will rise about 5 more degrees.

3. Stove-top Method: We use a cast-iron grill pan for steaks when cooking steak the stove top. Turn the element to high and let the pan get good and hot. Melt Homemade Ghee (link to recipe) in hot pan.

4. Quickly sear the steaks on each side then turn the heat under the pan down to medium-high. Continue frying the steaks for 2 or 3 minutes per side. When the internal temperature reaches 120F – 130 F (as described above), remove the steaks from the pan. Let rest for a few minutes before serving.

Yield: 4 servings

Nutritional Information:

- Total Calories/Serving (6 oz rib-eye): 498 *(calorie count for other cuts will vary slightly)*
- Total Carbs: 0g
- Total Fat: 36g
- Fiber: 0g
- Protein: 42g

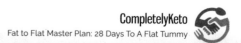

CompletelyKeto
Fat to Flat Master Plan: 28 Days To A Flat Tummy

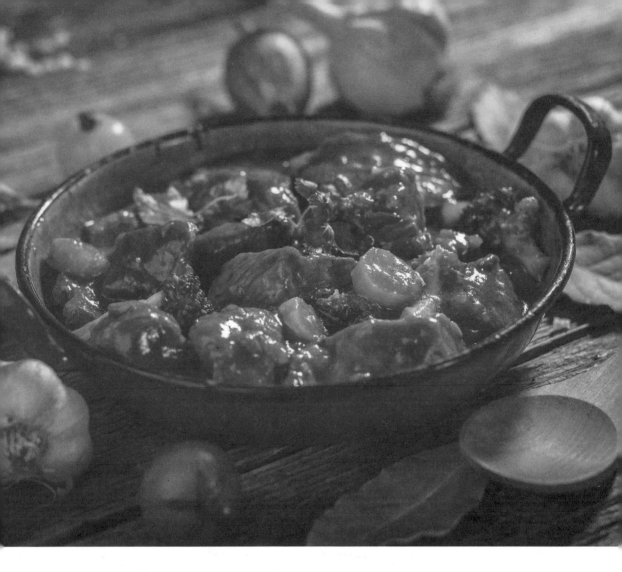

Lamb Stew

This recipe for lamb stew cooks up tender and juicy in less than an hour when you employ an Instant Pot.

Ingredients

- 2 T extra virgin olive oil
- 1 yellow cooking onion, cut into chunks
- 2 lb lamb shoulder, cut into chunks
- 1 C organic chicken (or beef) broth
- 1 tsp ground rosemary
- 1 tsp dried oregano
- ½ tsp dried thyme leaves
- ½ tsp xanthan gum
- Grinding of pink Himalayan salt and black pepper peppercorns

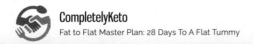

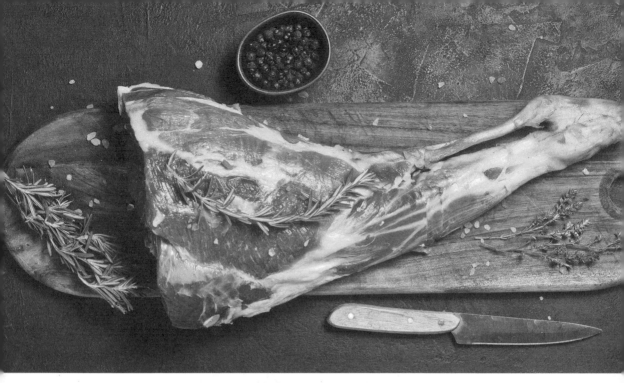

Preparation

1. Instant Pot Method: Set the Instant Pot to sauté. Allow the liner to heat for a few minutes then pour in 1 T of the olive oil. When it's hot, sauté the onion for three minutes until it softens slightly. Remove and set aside. Add remaining oil and sear the chunks of lamb on all sides. Do this in batches, if necessary. Remove seared meat from the pot, pour in the chicken (or beef) broth and deglaze the liner using a wooden spoon to scrape up the browned bits of meat from the bottom of the pan. Add the rosemary, oregano and thyme. Return the sautéed onion to the pot then add the browned lamb over-top. Secure the lid. Turn the steam valve to the correct position. Re-program the Instant Pot to the high pressure cooking setting and set the time for 35 minutes. When the time is up allow a natural release of the steam before opening the lid.

2. Oven Method: Pre-heat oven to 325 F. Heat enameled cast iron pot over medium high heat and sauté onion for a few minutes. Add the lamb and sauté, while stirring until the lamb is browned. Pour in the broth and add the spices and xanthan gum. Allow to simmer for a minute or two then place the covered casserole onto the middle rack of the pre-heated oven. Bake for 1-1 ½ hours until the lamb is tender. Serve with Cauliflower mash and enjoy.

Yield: 4 Servings

Nutritional Information:

- Total Calories/serving: 402
- Total Carbs: 3 g
- Fiber: 1 g
- Net Carbs: 2g
- Total Fat: 29 g
- Protein: 33 g

Nutritional Information:

- Calories/serving: 104
- Total Carbs: 6g
- Fiber: 1g
- Net carbs: 5g
- Total Fat: 6g
- Protein: 7g

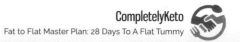

CompletelyKeto

Fat to Flat Master Plan: 28 Days To A Flat Tummy

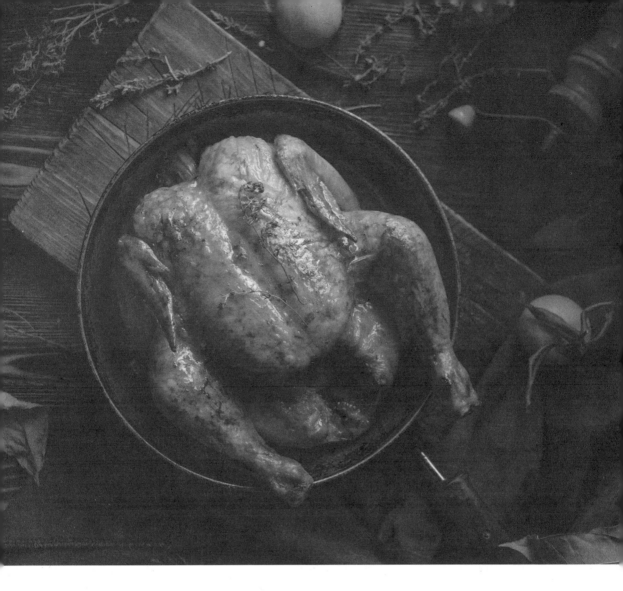

Easy Rustic Roasted Chicken

Roasted chicken dinner is a weekly event at our house.

Ingredients

- 5 to 6 lb chicken
- Fresh thyme and sage
- ½ cooking onion
- 1 T extra virgin olive oil
- 1 tsp garlic powder or garlic granules
- 1 tsp dried thyme
- Grinding of pink Himalayan salt and black peppercorns
- ½ C chicken broth
- ½ C coconut cream

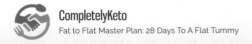

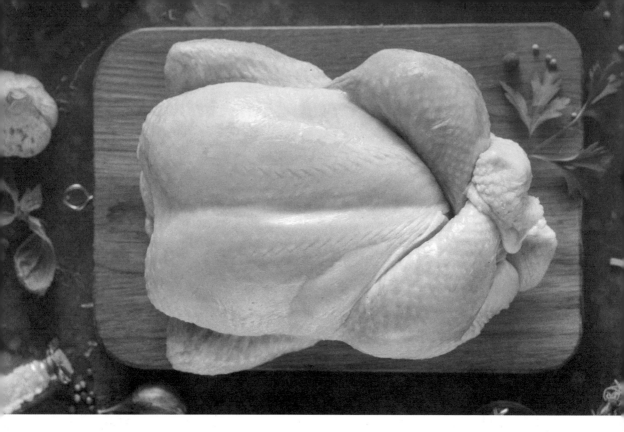

Preparation

1. Pre-heat oven to 500 F

2. Rinse chicken and pat dry.

3. Insert cooking onion and herb sprigs into the chicken cavity.

4. Place chicken in roasting pan. Coat the outside of the bird with the olive oil and sprinkle on the garlic powder, dried thyme, salt and pepper.

5. Place the roasting pan with the chicken on the middle rack of the pre-heated oven and immediately turn the oven heat down to 350 F. Roast for approximately 1 - 1 ½ hours or until the internal temperature reaches 165 F. Baste chicken with the pan juices half way through the roasting period.

6. Remove chicken from the pan and allow to rest while you make the gravy.

7. Deglaze the pan with the broth, scraping the browned bits off the bottom of the pan and stirring them into the broth. Add the coconut cream and stir while the gravy comes to a boil. Lower the heat and simmer the gravy for a few minutes while the gravy thickens.

8. Drizzle a bit of gravy over the carved chicken on each plate before serving.

Yield: 4 Servings

Nutritional Information:

- Total Calories/serving: 268
- Total Carbs: 3g
- Fiber: 1g
- Net Carbs: 2g
- Total Fat: 22g
- Protein: 26g

CompletelyKeto
Fat to Flat Master Plan: 28 Days To A Flat Tummy

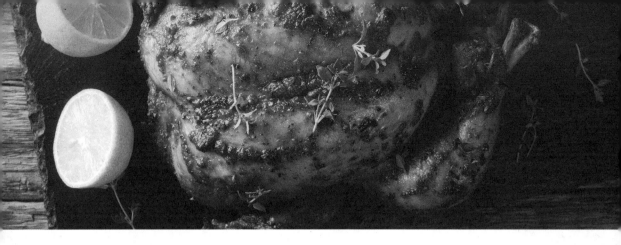

Citrus Thyme Roasted Chicken

Citrus pairs well with chicken and adds some zing to a family pleasing meal. Easily prepped, this main course dinner item goes into the oven quickly and leaves you time to organize your side dishes. You may even get to put your feet up for a few minutes before it's time to serve!

Ingredients

- 4 ½ lb – 5 lb whole chicken
- Grinding of pink Himalayan salt and black peppercorns
- 1 lemon, quartered
- 1 1/2 T thyme leaves
- 3 T freshly squeezed lemon juice
- 2 T extra-virgin olive oil

Preparation

1. Pre-heat oven to 500 F.
2. Pat chicken dry and season the cavity with salt and pepper. Tuck the lemon quarters inside the cavity.
3. Mix the lemon juice and olive oil and baste the outside of the chicken with this mixture. Sprinkle on the thyme leaves and season the outside of the chicken with salt and pepper.
4. Place the chicken in a roasting pan and set the pan on the middle rack of the pre-heated oven. Immediately turn the oven heat down to 350 F. Roast the chicken for 15 minutes then check the internal temperature. The chicken is done when the internal temperature reaches 165 F. Check both the light and dark meat areas when determining the internal temperature. Continue roasting if it needs a bit more time.
5. Allow the chicken to rest for a few minutes before carving and serving.

Yield: 4 Servings

Nutritional Information:

- Calories/serving: 443
- Total Carbs: 2g
- Fiber: 1g
- Net carbs: 1g
- Total Fat: 29g
- Protein: 28g

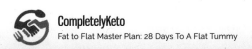

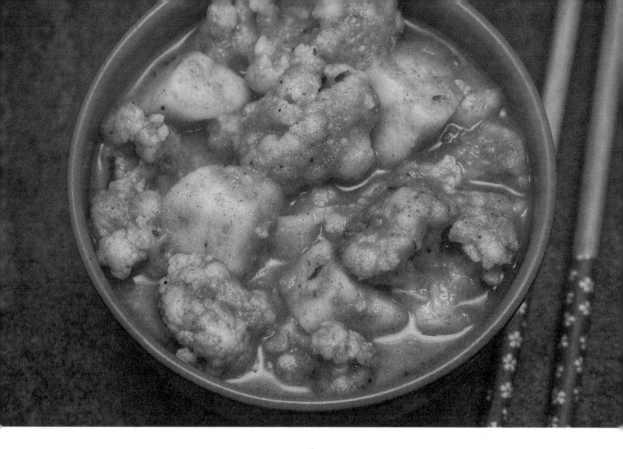

Coconut Cauliflower Chicken Curry

This meal is perfect for a busy week-day night when you have to eat and run. It will satisfy your appetite and have you out the door once more, in no time at all!

Ingredients

For the red curry sauce:

- 1 T extra virgin olive oil
- 1 tsp onion powder
- 2 tsp curry powder
- 1 garlic clove, minced or pushed through a press
- 1 medium tomato, medium dice
- 1 can full fat coconut milk
- ½ tsp dried chili flake
- Grinding of pink Himalayan salt, to taste

For the chicken and cauliflower:

- 1 T extra virgin olive oil
- 1 lb boneless/skinless chicken thighs, cut into bite-sized pieces
- 1 C cauliflower, cut into bite-sized florets
- 1 T fresh flat leaf parsley (or cilantro), chopped

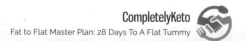
CompletelyKeto

Fat to Flat Master Plan: 28 Days To A Flat Tummy

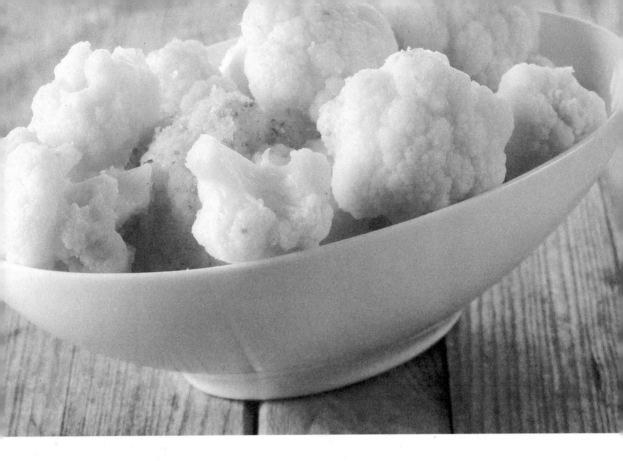

Preparation

For the red curry sauce:

6. Heat the oil in a saucepan over medium heat. Add the onion powder, curry powder, chili flakes and garlic.

7. Sauté for ½ minute. Add the remaining sauce ingredients and leave over heat, while stirring, until warmed through. Transfer to a blender or food processor and pulse until smooth. Set aside.

For the chicken and cauliflower:

8. Heat olive oil in a heavy bottomed skillet over medium high heat. Sauté the chicken until it is no longer pink in color. Stir in the cauliflower florets and curry sauce. Adjust the heat so the sauce is just simmering, Cover with a tight fitting lid and simmer for about 10 minutes or until the chicken reaches 165F and the cauliflower is soft and cooked.

9. Divide the cauliflower/chicken mixture between 4 wide bowls and serve, garnished with parsley (or cilantro).

Yield: 4 servings

Nutritional Information:

- Calories/serving: 439
- Net carbs: 4g
- Total Carbs: 5g
- Total Fat: 38g
- Fiber: 1g
- Protein: 19g

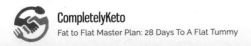

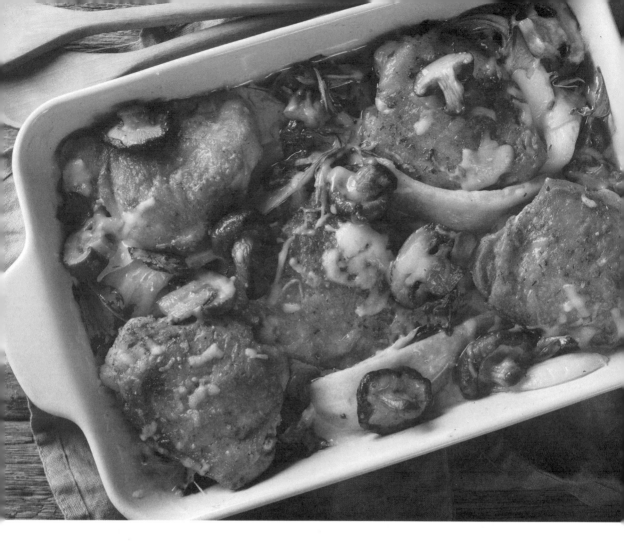

Chicken Thighs and Baby Bok Choy

I like to serve this rustic meal straight from the skillet. With minimal effort this recipe comes together quickly.

Ingredients

- 1 T extra-virgin olive oil
- 1 tsp garlic powder
- 1 tsp ground ginger
- 1 tsp Chinese five spice
- Grinding of black peppercorns
- 4 chicken thighs, skin on/bone in
- ¼ C Speed Keto Teriyaki Sauce
- 4 small baby bok choy heads, cut in half length-wise
- 1 C sliced mushrooms
- 2 green onions (scallions), thinly sliced

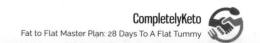

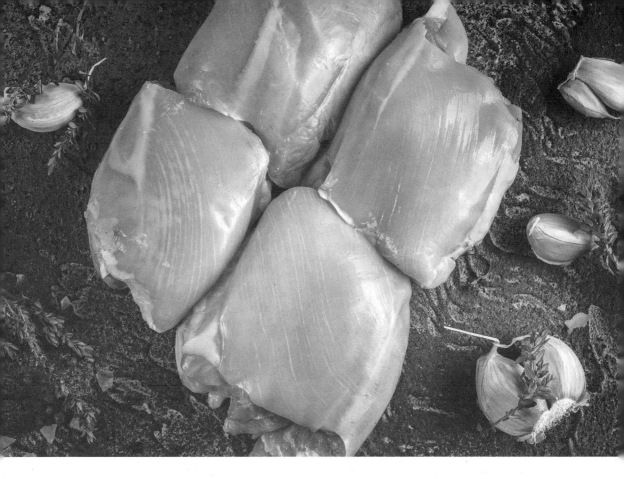

Preparation

1. Preheat oven to 375 F

2. Arrange chicken in an oven proof skillet, brush with olive oil and sprinkle garlic powder, ginger, five spice and pepper evenly over-top.

3. Drizzle Teriyaki sauce over the chicken and place the skillet on the middle rack of the pre-heated oven. Bake for 30 – 40 minutes or until the internal temperature of the thighs reaches 165 F.

4. Run the chicken under the broiler for a few minutes to crisp up the skin.

5. Heat remaining oil in a skillet and sauté mushrooms for a few minutes until a nice golden brown in color. Keep warm.

6. Steam the bok choy for a few minutes so it is cooked but still has some crunch. This won't take long. Tuck the bok choy around the chicken in the skillet and sprinkle the mushrooms over-top. Garnish with the sliced green onions. Serve from the skillet at the table.

Yield: 4 Servings

Nutritional Information:

- Calories/serving: 296
- Net carbs: 2g
- Total Carbs: 4g
- Total Fat: 23g
- Fiber: 2g
- Protein: 18g

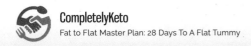

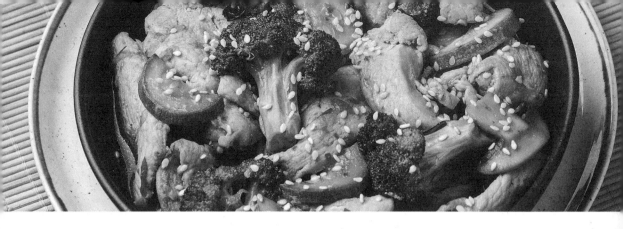

Simple Keto Hunan Chicken

Ingredients

- 2 T extra-virgin olive oil
- 1 lb boneless, skinless chicken breasts, cut into bite-sized chunks
- 2 C broccoli florets
- 1 small zucchini, cut into wheels then halved
- 2 garlic cloves
- ½ C broth (chicken or vegetable)
- 2 T gluten free tamari sauce
- 1 T keto fish sauce
- 2 tsp rice vinegar (unseasoned)
- 2 tsp Homemade Fermented Hot Sauce, or other keto-style (no sugar) hot sauce
- ¼ tsp xanthan gun

Preparation

1. Heat 1 T of the oil in a wok over medium high heat. Add chicken and stir-fry about 4-5 minutes until cooked (internal temperature of chicken chunks reaches 165 F). Remove and keep warm.

2. Heat remaining oil and add the broccoli florets. Stir fry for 3 minutes then add the zucchini, garlic. Stir-fry for minute more.

3. Whisk broth, tamari sauce, fish sauce, rice vinegar and xanthan gum.

4. Add the chicken chunks back into the wok and pour the broth mixture over-top. Stir fry for a few more minutes while the broth mixture thickens then remove from heat, divide into 4 servings and serve while hot.

Yield: 4 Servings

Nutritional Information:

- Calories/serving: 233
- Net carbs: 3g
- Total Carbs: 4g
- Total Fat: 8g
- Fiber: 1g
- Protein: 29g

CompletelyKeto
Fat to Flat Master Plan: 28 Days To A Flat Tummy
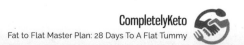

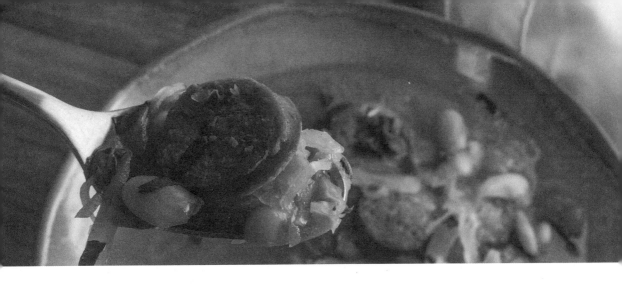

Turkey Keilbasa Oktoberfest Stew

Ingredients

- 1 T extra virgin olive oil
- ½ yellow cooking onion, medium dice
- 2 C shredded cabbage
- ¼ tsp crushed caraway seeds
- 2 garlic cloves, minced or pushed through a press
- 3 ½ C beef broth
- 1 T apple cider vinegar
- 10 oz smoked turkey kielbasa sausage, cut into bite-sized pieces
- 1 C Homemade Sauerkraut
- Grinding of pink Himalayan salt and black peppercorns, to taste
- Fresh parsley for garnish, optional

Preparation

1. Heat oil in heavy bottomed pot over medium high heat and sauté onions until translucent and golden in color.

2. Add cabbage, caraway, garlic, broth and vinegar. Simmer the stew until the cabbage is soft and cooked.

3. Add the kielbasa and sauerkraut. Simmer for 5 minutes more. Ladle the stew into 4 separate bowls, correct flavor with salt and pepper and garnish with parsley, if desired. Enjoy!

Yield: 4 Servings

Nutritional Information:

- Calories/serving: 328
- Net carbs: 5g
- Total Carbs: 7g
- Total Fat: 25g
- Fiber: 2g
- Protein: 16g

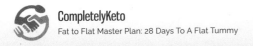

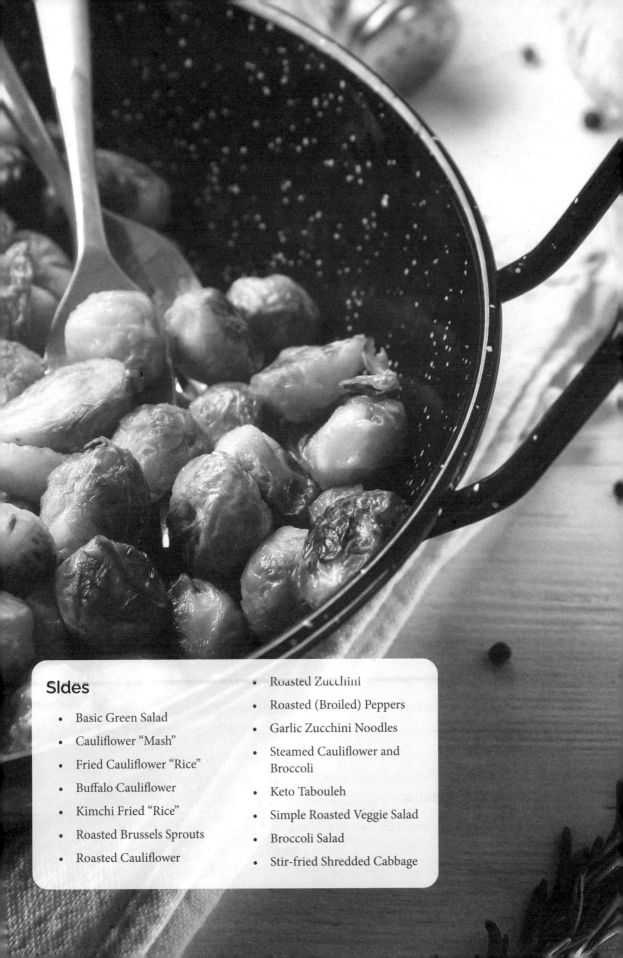

Sides

- Basic Green Salad
- Cauliflower "Mash"
- Fried Cauliflower "Rice"
- Buffalo Cauliflower
- Kimchi Fried "Rice"
- Roasted Brussels Sprouts
- Roasted Cauliflower
- Roasted Zucchini
- Roasted (Broiled) Peppers
- Garlic Zucchini Noodles
- Steamed Cauliflower and Broccoli
- Keto Tabouleh
- Simple Roasted Veggie Salad
- Broccoli Salad
- Stir-fried Shredded Cabbage

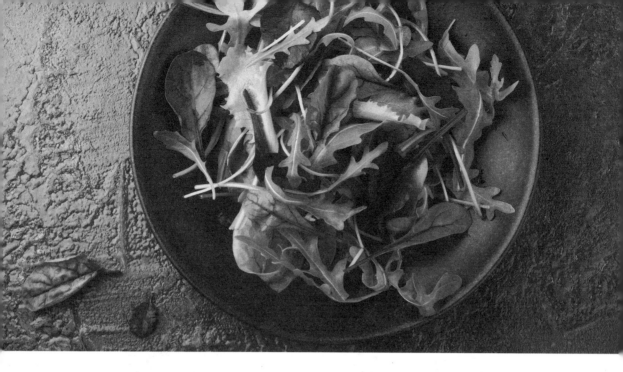

Basic Green Salad

Here's a basic green salad for everyday use. Dress it up with a few additions or dress it down as you wish. Bags of mixed greens available in the produce section of the grocery store make it easy to enjoy a good salad whenever you want!

Ingredients

- 2 C mixed greens
- 2 C romaine lettuce pieces
- ¼ C spring onion, thin slices
- ½ C cucumber, medium dice
- ¼ C fresh oregano leaves, chopped
- ¼ C extra-virgin olive oil
- 2 T lemon juice

Preparation

1. Toss mixed greens, romaine lettuce, spring onion, cucumber and oregano together.
2. Whisk olive oil and lemon juice then drizzle the dressing over the green salad. Toss again and serve.

Yield: 4 servings

Nutritional Information:

- Total Calories/serving: 129
- Total Carbs: 1 g
- Fiber: 1 g
- Total Fat: 14 g
- Protein: 1 g

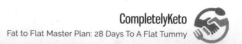

CompletelyKeto

Fat to Flat Master Plan: 28 Days To A Flat Tummy

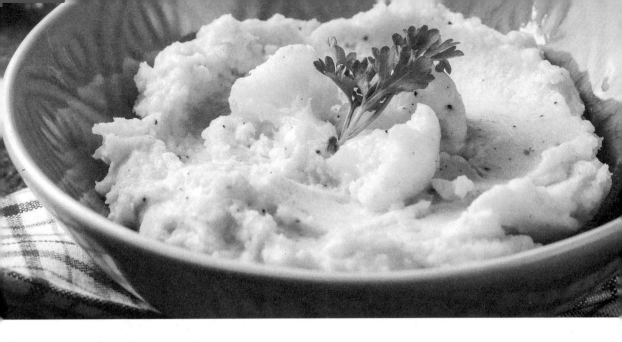

Cauliflower Mash

For creamy cauliflower mash you will need to take care when squeezing the excess moisture out of the steamed cauliflower. It's a bit of a messy process but the end result is worth your effort. The mash will be creamier and thicker ... just the way you like it!

Ingredients

- 1 head of cauliflower, cut into florets
- 3 T extra-virgin olive oil
- Grinding of black pepper corns and pink Himalayan salt, to taste

Preparation

1. Pre-heat oven to 375 F.
2. Steam cauliflower over boiling water until very tender. Transfer cooked cauliflower to a deep bowl. Fold a few sections of paper towel and place on top of the cauliflower.
3. Using paper towel squeeze as much excess moisture as possible out of the florets by pressing down on them. The moisture will wick upwards into the paper towel. Don't worry if the cauliflower falls apart during this process.
4. Mash the cauliflower using an emersion blender. Don't be afraid that the mash will get gluey by over-processing. It's the starch in potatoes that does that and since there's no starch in cauliflower, you don't have to worry! Stir olive oil into the mashed cauliflower. Serve and enjoy!

Yield: 4 Servings

Nutritional Information:

- Total Calories/Serving: 155
- Total Carbs: 11g
- Fiber: 5g
- Net Carbs: 6g
- Total Fat: 10g
- Protein: 4g

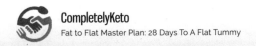

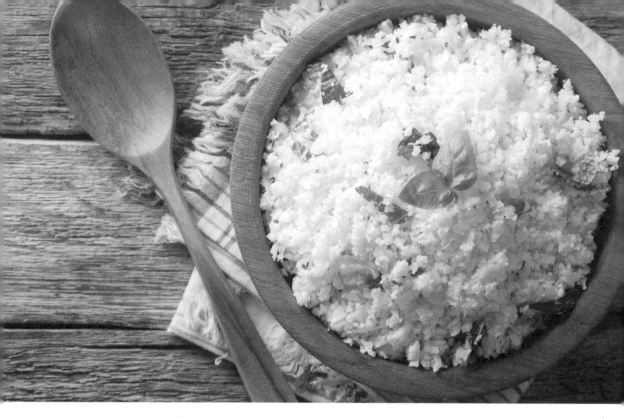

Fried Cauliflower "Rice"

You can use a variety of different spices and herbs to create different flavor profiles for this tasty "rice". It's a versatile side-dish that works well with many different entrées.

Ingredients

- 2 T extra virgin olive oil (or coconut oil)
- 2 C cauliflower, chopped in blender, grated with box grater or purchase "rice" fresh or frozen
- ¼ C onion, fine dice
- 2 garlic cloves, minced

Preparation

1. Melt oil in a wok or heavy skillet over medium/high heat.
2. Sauté onion for 3 minutes or until soft. Add minced garlic and sauté for one minute more.
3. Add cauliflower and stir-fry for about 4 or 5 minutes until the rice is soft and cooked through. Remove from heat and serve immediately.

Yield: 4 servings (½ C each)

Nutritional Information:

- Total Calories/serving: 86
- Total Carbs: 4g
- Fiber: 1g
- Net Carbs: 3g
- Total Fat: 8g
- Protein: 1g

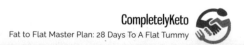
CompletelyKeto
Fat to Flat Master Plan: 28 Days To A Flat Tummy

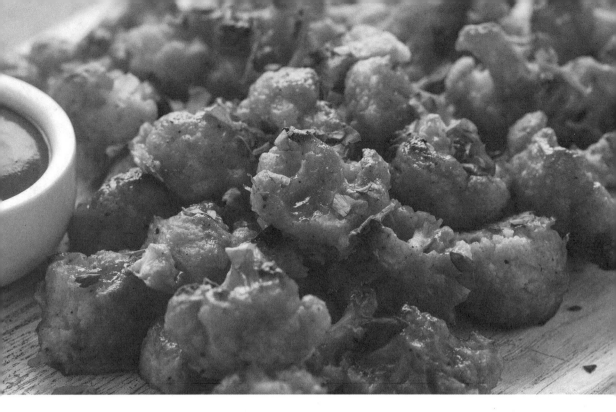

Buffalo Cauliflower

Ingredients

- ¼ C Fermented Hot Pepper Sauce
- 2 T extra virgin olive oil
- ½ tsp smoked paprika
- 2 garlic cloves, minced or pushed through a press
- Grinding of pink Himalayan salt and black peppercorns
- 4 C cauliflower florets

Preparation

1. Pre-heat oven to 375 F.
2. Mix together hot sauce, oil, paprika, garlic, salt and pepper.
3. Add florets and toss until the florets are evenly coated.
4. Place florets in non-stick baking pan and bake, on the middle rack of the pre-heated oven for 25 minutes. Serve while hot and enjoy.

Yield: 4 Servings

Nutritional Information:

- Calories/serving: 130
- Net carbs: 3g
- Total Carbs: 6g
- Total Fat: 12g
- Fiber: 3g
- Protein: 2g

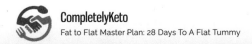

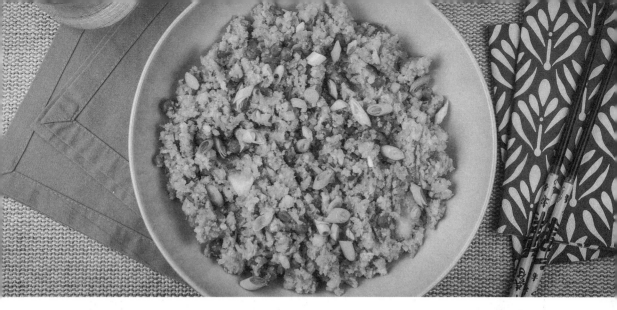

Kimchi Fried "Rice"

Ingredients

- 4 C cauliflower florets (or use 4 C frozen cauliflower rice)
- 2 T plus extra-virgin olive oil
- 2/3 C Keto Kimchi
- 2 garlic cloves, minced or pushed through a press
- 1 T fresh ginger root, minced
- 2 T kimchi juice
- 1 T gluten free tamari sauce
- Grinding of pink Himalayan salt and black peppercorns, to taste
- 1 green onion, optional (for garnish)

Preparation

1. Place cauliflower florets in high speed blender (or food processor) and pulse a few times until florets are cut into rice-sized bits.

2. Heat 2 T of the oil in a wok over medium high heat. Add the cauliflower rice, kimchi, garlic, kimchi juice, ginger and tamari sauce.

3. Stir-fry for about 5 minutes until the cauliflower rice softens and is cooked and the kimchi is heated through. Season mixture with a grinding of salt and pepper. Garnish with thinly sliced green onion, if desired, and serve.

Yield: 4 Servings (¾ C/serving)

Nutritional Information:

- Calories/serving: 122
- Total Carbs: 8g
- Fiber: 3g
- Net carbs: 5g
- Total Fat: 9g
- Protein: 5g

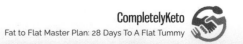

CompletelyKeto
Fat to Flat Master Plan: 28 Days To A Flat Tummy

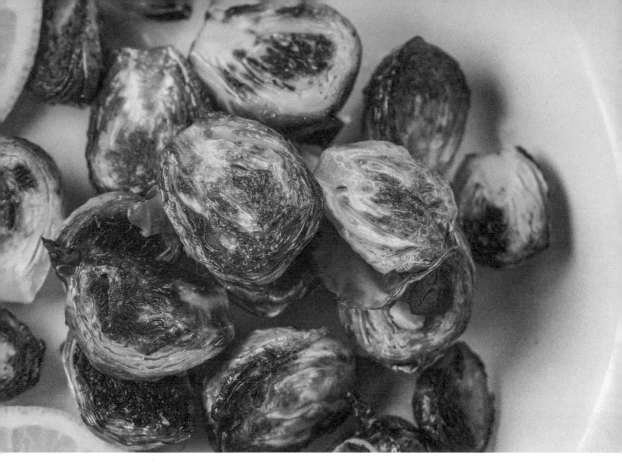

Roasted Brussels Sprouts

Ingredients

- 2 C Brussels sprouts, cut in half
- 1 T extra-virgin olive oil
- Grinding of pink Himalayan salt and black peppercorns

Preparation

1. Toss Brussels sprouts with oil and season with salt and pepper.
2. Air Fryer Method: Spread out on tray of air fryer. Program for 20 min. at 400 F. Give the tray a shake half way through the roasting period.
3. Oven Method: Preheat oven to 350 F. Spread Brussels sprouts out on a rimmed baking sheet and place on the middle rack of the pre-heated oven. Roast for 20 minutes until done to your liking.

Yield: 4 Servings (½ C/serving)

Nutritional Information:

- Calories/serving: 52
- Net carbs: 2g
- Total Carbs: 4g
- Total Fat: 4g
- Fiber: 2g
- Protein: 2g

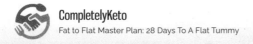

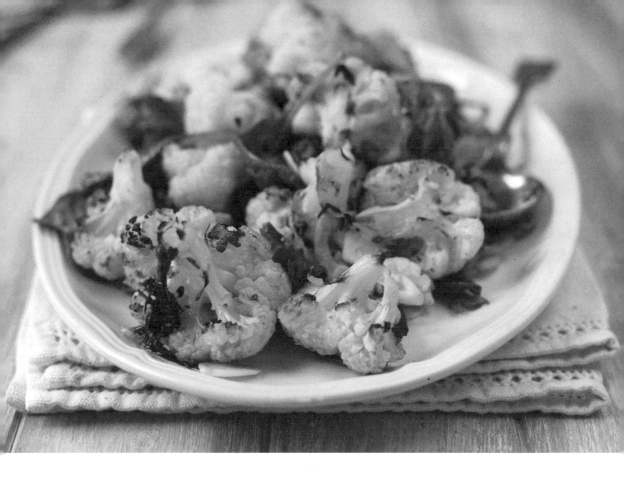

Roasted Cauliflower

Ingredients

- 2 C cauliflower florets
- 1 T extra-virgin olive oil
- Grinding of pink Himalayan salt and black peppercorns

Preparation

1. Toss florets with oil and season with salt and pepper.

2. Air Fryer Method: Spread out on tray of air fryer. Program for 15 minutes at 400 F. Give the tray a shake half way through the roasting period.

3. Oven Method: Preheat oven to 350 F. Spread florets out on a rimmed baking sheet and place on the middle rack of the pre-heated oven. Roast for 15 – 20 minutes until done to your liking.

Yield: 4 Servings (½ C/serving)

Nutritional Information:

- Calories/serving: 45
- Net carbs: 2g
- Total Carbs: 4g
- Total Fat: 4g
- Fiber: 2g
- Protein: 1g

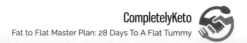

CompletelyKeto

Fat to Flat Master Plan: 28 Days To A Flat Tummy

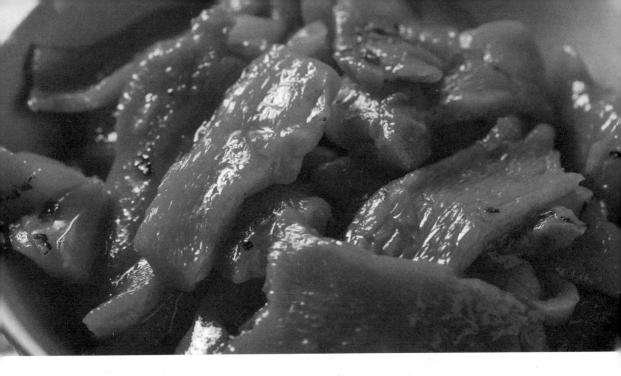

Roasted (Broiled) Peppers

Some people find it difficult to digest the skin on peppers. If this is something you deal with try broiling peppers. Broiling makes skin removal very easy. Peppers deepen and at the same time mellow in flavor when treated this way.

You can also buy jars of roasted peppers that have no extra sugars added and you may find this to be the easiest option of all!

Ingredients

- 2 bell peppers, seeded and cut lengthwise into pieces
- ½ T extra-virgin olive oil

Preparation

1. Toss with oil and spread pepper pieces out on a rimmed baking sheet lined with foil. Turn broiler on and place baking sheet beneath the broiler element. Broil until the pepper skins blacken and blister, remove from oven.

2. Wrap foil up and around the peppers and seal into a packet. The resulting steam from the hot peppers inside the packet will work to loosen the skins within a few minutes.

3. Open packet and slip the charred skins off the roasted pepper pieces. The roasted peppers are now ready to use in a variety of recipes or enjoy them as is!

Yield: 4 Servings (1/2 pepper/serving)

Nutritional Information:

- Calories/serving: 35
- Total Carbs: 4g
- Fiber: 1g
- Net carbs: 3g
- Total Fat: 2g
- Protein: 1g

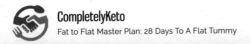

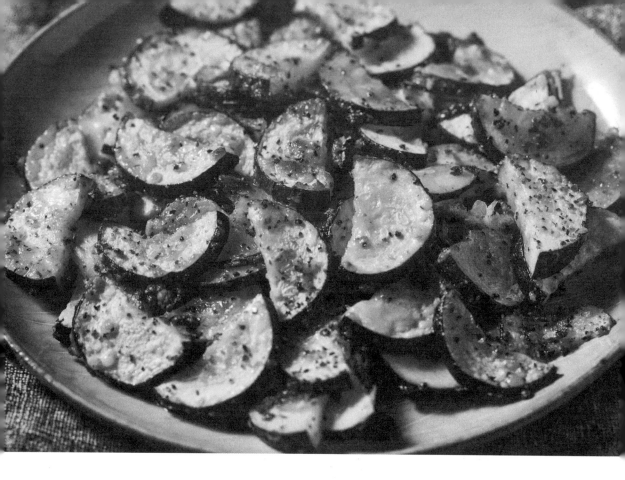

Roasted Zucchini

Ingredients

- 2 small zucchini, sliced into sticks or wheels
- 1 T extra virgin olive oil
- Grinding of pink Himalayan salt and black peppercorns, to taste

Preparation

4. Toss zucchini with oil and season with salt and pepper.
5. Air Fryer Method: Spread out on tray of air fryer. Program for 12 minutes at 400 F. Give the tray a shake half way through the roasting period.
6. Oven Method: Preheat oven to 350 F. Spread zucchini out on a rimmed baking sheet and place on the middle rack of the pre-heated oven. Roast for 15 – 20 minutes until done to your liking.

Yield: 4 Servings

Nutritional Information:

- Calories/serving: 43
- Net carbs: 1g
- Total Carbs: 2g
- Total Fat: 4g
- Fiber: 1g
- Protein: 1g

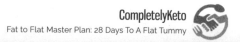

CompletelyKeto
Fat to Flat Master Plan: 28 Days To A Flat Tummy

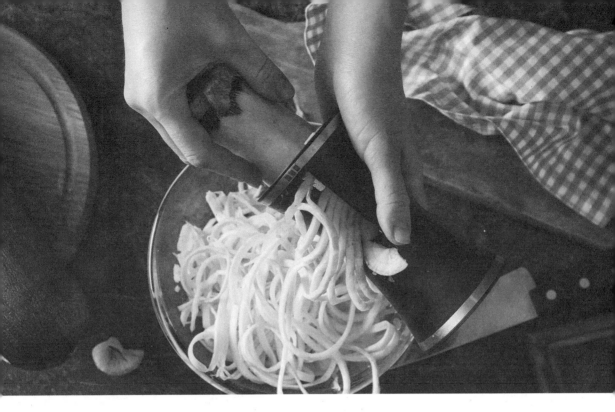

Garlic Zucchini Noodles

Ingredients

- 3 zucchini, small size
- 2 cloves of garlic, minced
- Grinding of salt and pepper, to taste

Preparation

1. Wash zucchini, pat dry and trim the ends. Spiralize into noodles. If you don't have a spiralizer slice zucchini lengthwise into very thin slices. Lay each slice flat and cut, lengthwise into flat fettuccini noodle style strips about 1/3 " wide. You will have about 5 – 6 cups of "veggie pasta" when done.

2. Melt ghee in a wok or flat-bottomed skillet over medium high heat.

3. Add minced garlic and cook, stirring until the garlic becomes translucent.

4. Add the zucchini noodles and continue stir-frying until the zucchini is softens and is cooked. This will only take a few minutes. Careful not to over-cook or the noodles will become mushy. Serve immediately

Yield: 4 servings

Nutritional Information:

- Total Calories/serving: 50
- Total Carbs: 3 g
- Fiber: 1 g
- Net Carbs: 2g
- Total Fat: 4 g
- Protein: 1 g

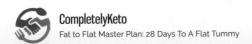

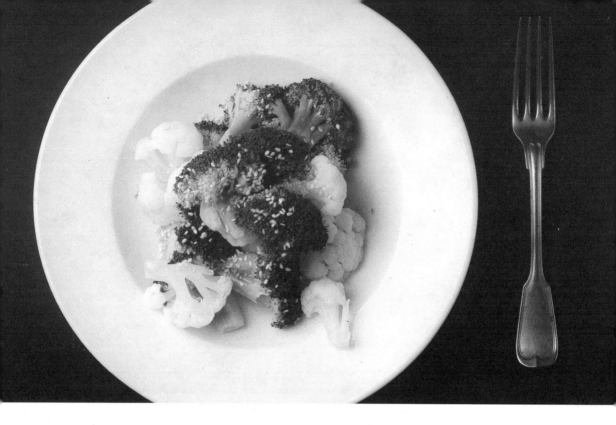

Steamed Cauliflower and Broccoli

Steamed lightly and served with ghee melting over-top this combo can accompany a variety of entrees. These veggie florets feel right at home next to either fish or meat.

Ingredients

- 3 C broccoli florets
- 3 C cauliflower florets
- 2 T ghee
- Salt and pepper to taste

Preparation

1. Fill the bottom of a large pot with about 2" of water.

2. Place steamer over the water put in the cauliflower and broccoli florets. Cover the pot with a tight fitting lid and steam over medium-high heat. Steam for 5-7 minutes until, the florets are tender but still slightly crunchy.

3. Serve immediately with butter melting over-top!

Yield: Serves 4

Nutritional Information:

- Total Calories/serving: 95
- Total Carbs: 8 g
- Fiber: 4 g
- Total Fat: 6 g
- Protein: 4 g

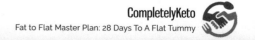

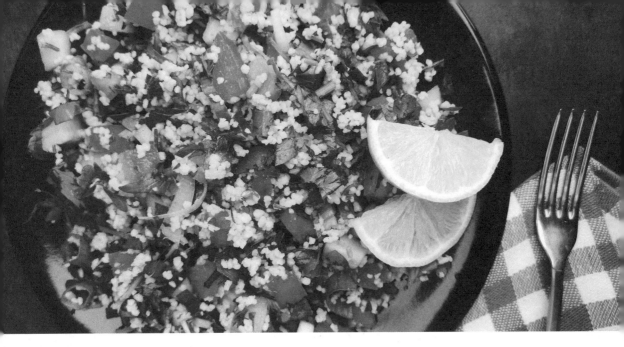

Keto Tabouleh

Tabouleh salad traditionally is made with bulgur but I've elected to use hemp hearts. However, there's more than one way to make a keto version of this classic. You can also easily substitute cauliflower rice that's been cooked and chilled for a lighter, and equally delicious outcome.

Ingredients

- 1 C, flat leaf parsley
- ¾ C hemp hearts
- 2 T fresh mint
- 1 medium tomato, small dice
- 2 green onions, thinly sliced
- 1 garlic clove, minced or pushed through a press
- 2 T extra-virgin olive oil
- 2 T freshly squeezed lemon juice

Preparation

1. In a glass bowl mix together the parsley, hemp hearts, mint, tomato and green onion.
2. Whisk garlic, oil and lemon juice. Pour over hemp heart mixture and toss. Serve immediately at room temperature or chill for an hour in the fridge, if preferred.

Yield: 4 servings (½ C/serving)

Nutritional Information:

- Calories/serving: 251
- Net carbs: 2g
- Total Carbs: 4g
- Total Fat: 22g
- Fiber: 2g
- Protein: 11g

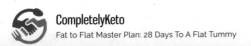

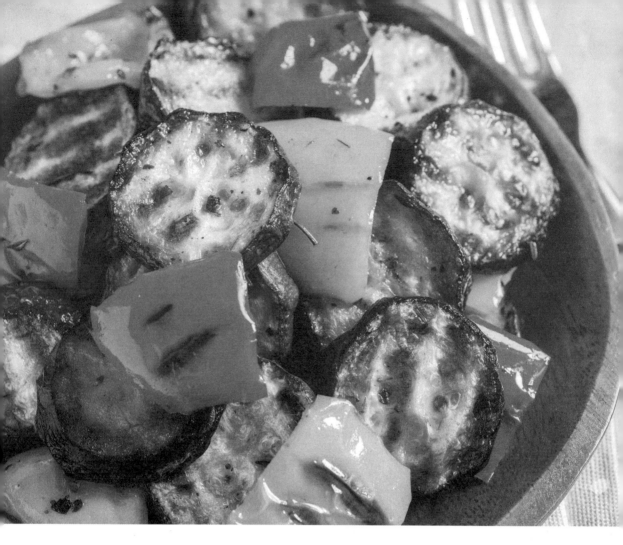

Simple Roasted Veggie Salad

Ingredients

- 1 full recipe of Roasted Zucchini
- 1 full recipe of Roasted Peppers
- 1 tsp dried thyme
- 2 T Vinaigrette

Preparation

1. In a glass bowl mix together all ingredients. Divide into 4 servings and enjoy!

Yield: 4 Servings

Nutritional Information:

- Calories/serving: 258
- Net carbs: 4g
- Total Carbs: 6g
- Total Fat: 24g
- Fiber: 2g
- Protein: 2g

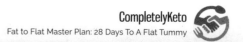

CompletelyKeto
Fat to Flat Master Plan: 28 Days To A Flat Tummy

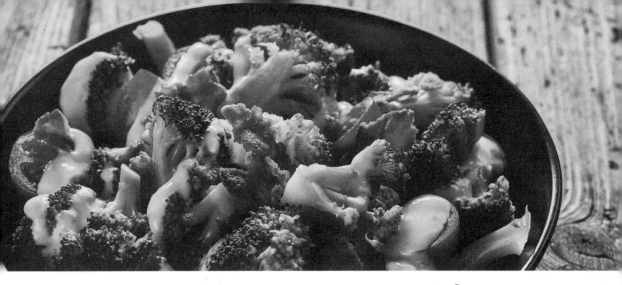

Broccoli Salad

Ingredients

- 4 C broccoli, chopped into bite-sized florets
- 8 cherry tomatoes, cut in half
- 2 red radishes, thinly sliced
- ¼ C red onion, thinly sliced
- ½ C full fat Greek yogurt
- ½ T Dijon mustard
- 1 T apple cider vinegar
- Few drops of liquid stevia, to taste
- 2 slices turkey bacon, fried until crisp and broken into pieces

Preparation

1. Steam broccoli for 3-4 minutes so it is partially cooked but still crispy and a nice bright green in color. Plunge florets immediately into water and ice to halt the cooking process immediately. Drain using a colander after a few minutes and set aside.

2. Make a dressing by whisking yogurt, mustard, and stevia (if using). Set aside.

3. Prepare the bacon, radish and red onion.

4. If necessary, pat the broccoli florets dry and divide between 4 salad bowls. Distribute the tomatoes, radish, red onion and bacon evenly between the bowls and drizzle the yogurt dressing over-top.

Yield: 4 Servings

Nutritional Information:

- Calories/serving: 87
- Net carbs: 7g
- Total Carbs: 10g
- Total Fat: 3g
- Fiber: 3g
- Protein: 9g

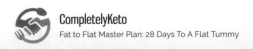

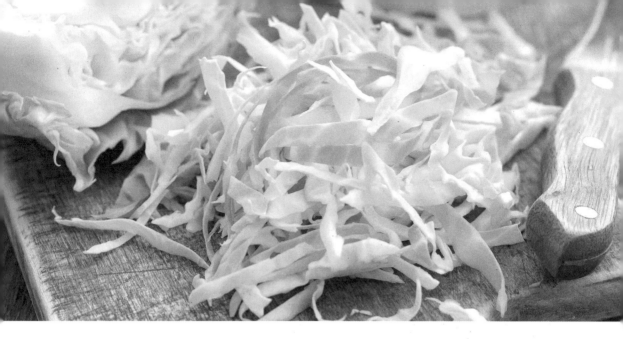

Stir-fried Shredded Cabbage

Make the recipe, as is, or substitute fermented peppers for the fresh red pepper listed in the ingredients. When fermented vegetables are used in any recipe another layer in interesting flavor is added to tantalize the taste buds.

Ingredients

- 2 T extra-virgin olive oil
- 2 C shredded Cabbage
- 1 C Homemade Keto Sauerkraut
- ½ onion, small dice
- ½ red bell pepper (or ¼ C roasted red pepper), seeded and cut into small slices
- ¼ C Fresh herbs of choice (if desired), roughly chopped

Preparation

1. Heat oil in a heavy bottomed wok over medium high heat. Add onion and stir fry for a few minutes.

2. Add shredded cabbage and Homemade Keto Sauerkraut. Continue to stir-fry for 4 - 5 more minutes until the cabbage is soft and cooked.

3. Add red pepper and stir fry for 2 more minutes. Stir in fresh herbs of choice and serve when the herbs have wilted.

Yield: 4 Servings

Nutritional Information:

- Total Calories/Serving: 132
- Total Carbs: 7g
- Fiber: 2g
- Net Carbs: 5g
- Total Fat: 11g
- Protein: 1g

CompletelyKeto
Fat to Flat Master Plan: 28 Days To A Flat Tummy

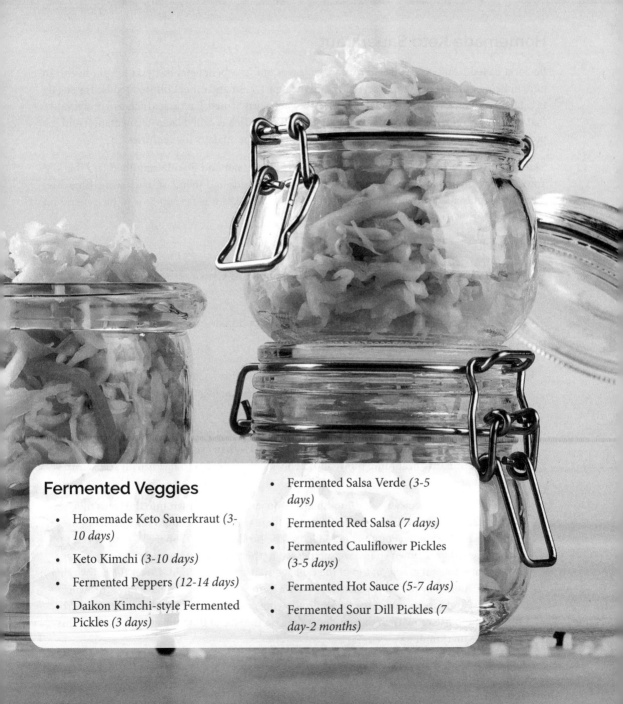

Fermented Veggies

- Homemade Keto Sauerkraut *(3-10 days)*
- Keto Kimchi *(3-10 days)*
- Fermented Peppers *(12-14 days)*
- Daikon Kimchi-style Fermented Pickles *(3 days)*
- Fermented Salsa Verde *(3-5 days)*
- Fermented Red Salsa *(7 days)*
- Fermented Cauliflower Pickles *(3-5 days)*
- Fermented Hot Sauce *(5-7 days)*
- Fermented Sour Dill Pickles *(7 day-2 months)*

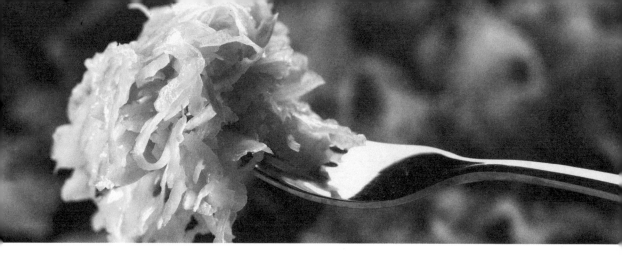

Homemade Keto Sauerkraut

Bacteria called lactobacillus lives on cabbage leaves and is a beneficial bacteria for gut health in human beings. This is the same bacteria found in yogurt, kefir and other cultured foods. The sugars in cabbage are converted into lactic acid when the cabbage is brined. Lactic acid acts as a preservative that stops harmful bacteria from developing in the kraut. This is called lacto-fermentation and is a process for preserving vegetables that's been in use by home-makers for centuries.

Sauerkraut is very easy to make; all you need is cabbage, salt and a wide-mouthed jar. That's it! You can customize it to your own taste by adding some seeds and then... sit back while time does the rest. I highly recommend you give it a try; homemade kraut is far superior to the sauerkraut available at the grocery store.

Ingredients

- 1medium sized head of cabbage, shredded (about 8-8 ½ C)
- 2 T pink Himalayan (or kosher) salt flakes
- 1 T mixed seeds (fennel, coriander, caraway, etc.), optional

Preparation

1. Remove large outer leaves (rinse and set aside for later use), Cut the cabbage in half, remove the core and shred into thin strips. Place the shredded cabbage into a big bowl and sprinkle the salt over-top.

2. Using clean hands massage the salt into the cabbage. Eventually the salt will cause the cabbage to become limp (more the texture of coleslaw than crisp raw cabbage).You will notice the mixture becoming moist and then watery. If you opt to flavor with seeds, mix them into the cabbage now.

3. Pack cabbage into a clean, wide-mouthed mason jar, pressing down into the jar as much as possible. Do not fill the jar up to the top as there will be more liquid released from the cabbage as it ferments. Pour any liquid left in the bowl over the cabbage. You will need to weigh the cabbage down so it stays submerged in the brine. Fold the reserved large outer leaf up and press it down on top of the cabbage so it acts as a weight. Cover the jar by tying on some muslin or folded cheesecloth or use a fermenting lid, if you have one. This will keep dust and insects out of the jar while allowing gas to escape as the kraut ferments. You may need to use more than one jar depending on the size of the cabbage you used for this batch of sauerkraut.

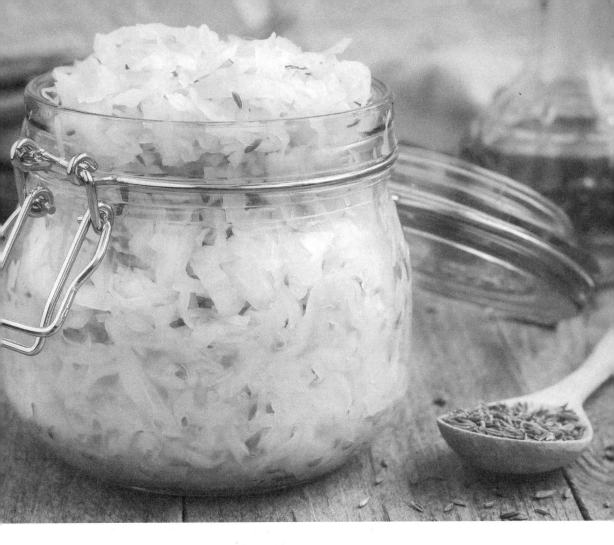

4. Store the jar(s) at room temperature, making sure to check on the amount of liquid a few times over the first 24 hours. Remove the cloth covering and press down into the jar so the shredded cabbage is covered by the liquid as much as possible. If the cabbage isn't completely submerged by the end of this time mix 1 tsp of salt into a cup of water and use this brine to cover the cabbage up completely. Replace the outer leaf and re-tie the cover back over-top the jar.

5. Allow the sauerkraut to ferment for a minimum of 3 days or up to 10 days. Keep out of direct sunlight and in a cool(ish) spot (65 F – 75 F). Check it daily to make sure the sauerkraut is staying submerged. Try a taste test after 3 days and keep doing this until the degree of sourness you prefer is reached. Once achieved simply refrigerate and use as desired. Jars of sauerkraut can be stored for months at 55F (cold area in your basement) or in your fridge, where it's easy to grab for daily use in keto recipes.

Yield: approx 12- 14 Servings (½ C/serving)

Nutritional Information:

- Calories/serving: 13
- Total Carbs: 3g
- Fiber: 1g

- Net carbs: 2g
- Total Fat: 0g
- Protein: 1g

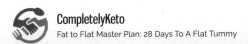

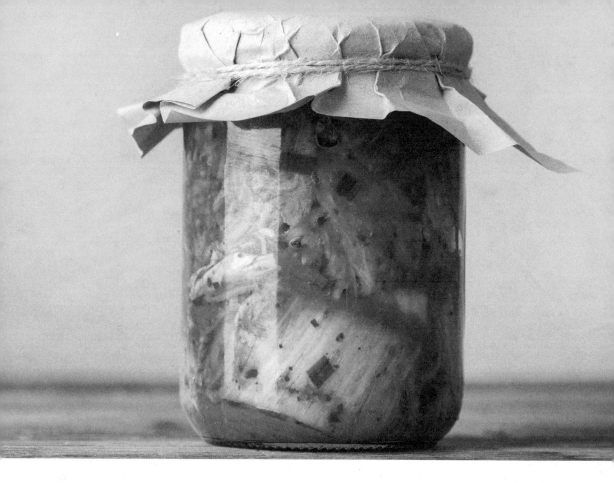

Keto Kimchi

Kimchi is similar to sauerkraut but uses a different type of cabbage and has a spicier, Korean flavored profile. Like kraut, kimchi is alive and infused with good, probiotic bacteria by the end of the fermenting period. Both these foods support the gut and promote good digestion and a healthy immune system. Goshugaru is a Korean chili powder traditionally used in Kimchi recipes and is usually found in Asian markets or online. If not easily available substitute pepper flakes which are hotter so you use less.

Ingredients

- 1 head of Nappa cabbage
- ½ daikon radish, sliced into thin matchsticks
- 4 green (spring) onions, sliced into 1" pieces
- 1/4 C salt flakes
- 4 cloves garlic, minced or pushed through a press
- 2 T fresh ginger, minced
- 5 T Korean chili powder, goshugaru (or 2 T red pepper flakes)
- 2 T nori flakes
- 2 T keto fish sauce (or miso)
- 4 or 5 drops liquid stevia, if desired

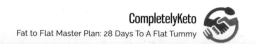

CompletelyKeto
Fat to Flat Master Plan: 28 Days To A Flat Tummy

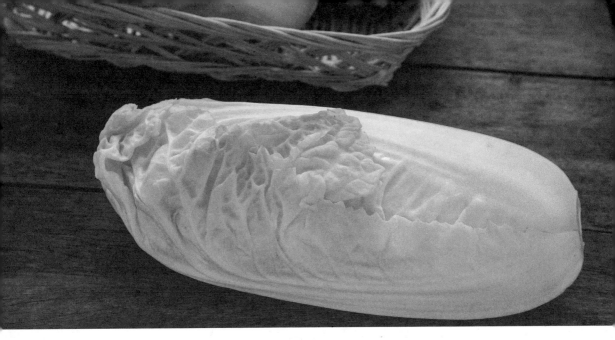

Preparation

1. Remove large outer leaves from the cabbage. Rinse, pat dry and reserve for later use. Quarter and core the cabbage before slicing each quarter into 1-inch chunks. Place chopped cabbage, daikon and green onions in a large bowl before sprinkling with salt. Massage into the cabbage mixture using your clean hands. Place a plate over-top the cabbage and weigh it down with something heavy. Let rest for 20-30 minutes. The salt will leach water from the cabbage mixture which will soften in the brine as it rests.

2. In a small bowl mix together the garlic, ginger, goshugaru, nori, fish sauce and stevia, if using. Stir into the brined cabbage mixture and mix well.

3. Place into a clean mason jar pressing the mixture down so that the released salty juices cover the cabbage mixture. If there isn't enough liquid add a bit more salted water. Fold a reserved outer leaf and place it over-top the cabbage in the jar. Press down using your fist so that the folded leaf weighs the cabbage down, keeping it covered in the brine. Leave room for the liquid that will accumulate as the kimchi ferments. Depending on the size of the cabbage you've used you may need to use more than one jar. Cover the jar(s) by tying on some muslin or folded cheesecloth. This will keep dust and insects out of the jar as the kimchi ferments. If you have a fermenting lid you can top the jar with this instead.

4. Allow the Kimchi to ferment for a minimum of 3 days. Keep out of direct sunlight and in a cool(ish) spot (65 F is perfect). Try a taste test after 3 days and keep doing this until the degree of tangy sourness you prefer is reached. Once achieved simply refrigerate and use as desired. You will find the kimchi continues to ferment but does so much more slowly in the fridge. The taste will mellow slightly after a few weeks.

Yield: 12 Servings (about 1/3 C/serving)

Nutritional Information:

- Calories/serving: 19
- Total Carbs: 4g
- Fiber: 1g
- Net carbs: 3g
- Total Fat: 0g
- Protein: 2g

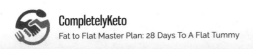

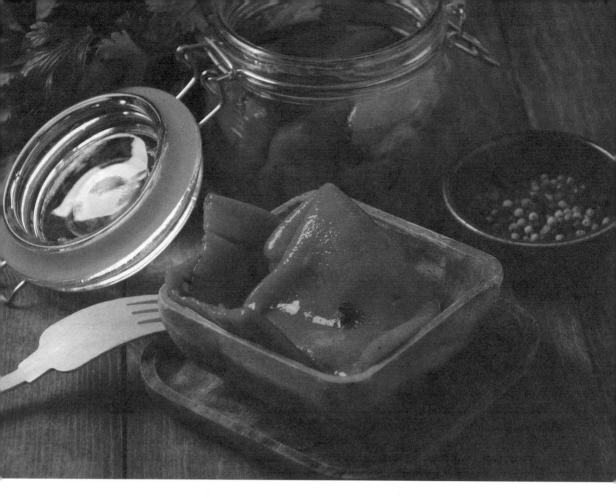

Fermented Peppers

The fermentation period for peppers is anywhere from 7-14 days so you may want to make up a batch in the first few days of the Fat to Flat Masterplan program. You may be able to buy pickled peppers at the grocery store but the flavor and nutritional make-up will be far superior when you make your own fermented peppers. I use Serrano peppers in this recipe but you can use the pepper variety that best suits your preference for heat level.

Use peppers from the loose bin at the grocery store as opposed to the super-washed ones that come pre-packaged. Often the aggressive washing process removes most of the healthy bacteria that live on the skin of a pepper (necessary for successful fermentation). Consider adding the powder from a probiotic supplement to hasten the fermentation process. You can also simply add a tablespoon of liquid from homemade sauerkraut for a similar affect.

Ingredients

- 1 T kosher salt flakes (or pink Himalayan salt flakes)
- 4 C filtered water
- Enough peppers of choice (jalapeno, Serrano, poblano, cayenne, banana, or bell) to fill a wide mouth pint sized Mason jar, about 3- 3 ½ C.
- 2 garlic cloves, peeled and left whole
- Powder from 1 capsule of probiotic (or 1 T sauerkraut liquid), optional

 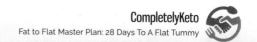

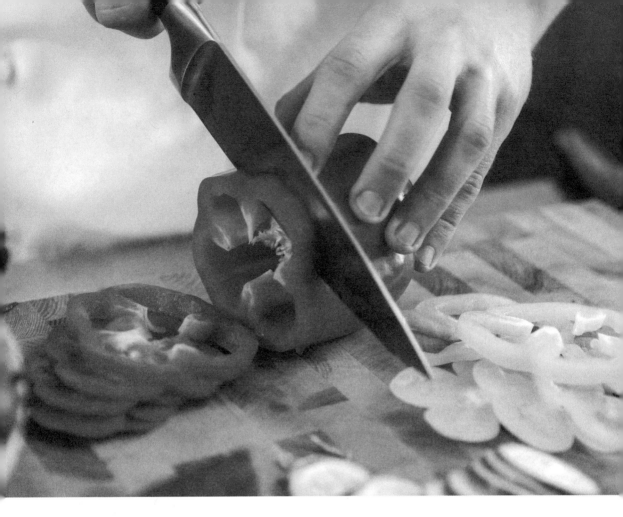

Preparation

1. Make brine by mixing salt flakes and water. Set aside.

2. Slice peppers (you can cut into rings or lengthwise depending on preference).

3. Remove seeds if desired. If you leave the seeds, the peppers will have more heat.

4. Pack peppers into wide mouth Mason jar. Put the peeled garlic cloves into the jar and pour the prepared brine over-top.

5. Place a glass fermentation weight on top of the peppers to keep them submerged. Remove any seeds that you find floating above the weight and add a <u>fermenting lid</u> to the jar.

6. Store in a cool, dark place for 5-10 days. Do a taste test on day 7 and then regularly after that until your preferred flavor emerges. Remove the fermenting lid and weight. Cover the jar with a <u>plastic storage lid</u> and store in the refrigerator.

Yield: 12 Servings

Nutritional Information:

- Calories/serving: 9
- Net carbs: 1g
- Total Carbs: 2g
- Total Fat: 0g
- Fiber: 1g
- Protein: 0g

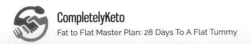

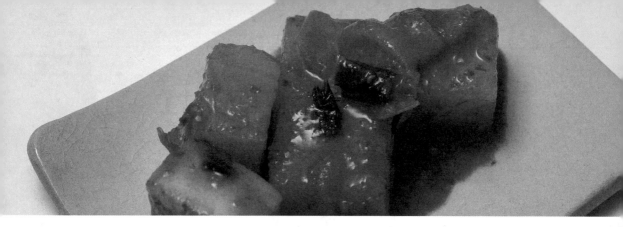

Daikon Kimchi-style Fermented Pickles

- The pungent smell of fermented daikon pickles (or daikon in the process of fermenting) is not pleasant to most people. However, if you give this recipe a try I think the end point; the fermented daikon pickle will surprise you with its tastiness.

- Ingredients

- 2 lb daikon radish, peeled and cut into small cubes or thin rounds

- 6 green onions (scallions), cut into 1" pieces

- 3 T minced fresh ginger root

- 4 garlic cloves, peeled and sliced thinly

- ¼ C goshugaru, Korean powdered chili (or substitute 2 T red pepper flakes)

- 2 T keto fish sauce

- 2 T pink Himalayan salt flakes or kosher salt flakes

Preparation

1. Combine all ingredients in a glass or ceramic bowl. Stir until all daikon surfaces are coated and an even mix of ingredients is achieved. Cover bowl and leave for 2 hours at room temperature. The daikon should release its juices during this time.

2. Pack mixture in to a clean, 1 qt., wide mouthed Mason jar. Press contents down as you pack the jar to remove air bubbles and to make room for all of the daikon mixture.

3. Use the remaining liquid in the bowl to cover the contents of the jar before placing the fermenting weight over-top. Seal, using a fermentation lid if you have one. If not use a regular lid but make sure to "burp" the jar daily to remove accumulated air and gases during the fermentation period.

4. Allow the daikon to ferment for 3 days then store in the refrigerator. As already mentioned, fermenting daikon has a very pungent odor. This is completely normal!

Yield: 12 servings

Nutritional Information:

- Calories/serving: 38
- Net carbs: 5g
- Total Carbs: 8g
- Total Fat: 0g
- Fiber: 3g
- Protein: 2g

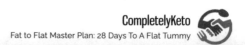

CompletelyKeto

Fat to Flat Master Plan: 28 Days To A Flat Tummy

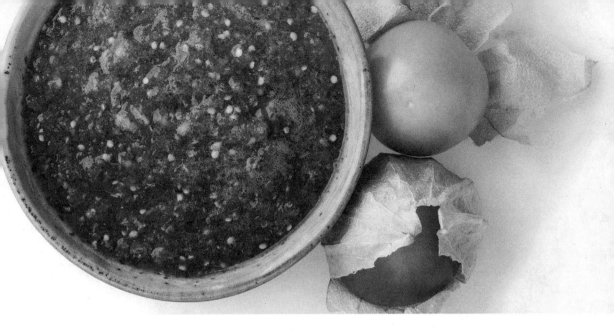

Fermented Salsa Verde

Fermented foods are eaten daily in this program. Salsa Verde pairs well with many meats and vegetable dishes and adds healthy probiotics to enhance gut health while adding zing to your meal. It isn't difficult to keep this fermented version of the condiment on hand in the fridge, as prep takes very little time. To speed up fermentation add the powder from in probiotic capsule.

Ingredients

- ¾ lb (12 oz) tomatillos, husk removed and quartered
- 3 medium sized jalapenos, stems removed, and cut in half
- 3 garlic cloves, peeled
- ½ small white onion, peeled and cut into chunks
- 1 C fresh cilantro
- 1 tsp ground coriander
- Juice from 1 lime
- 2 tsp pink Himalayan salt flakes

Preparation

1. Place all ingredients in high-speed blender or food processor. Pulse until a sauce forms. Transfer salsa to a clean, pint-sized, wide-mouthed mason jar(s) and seal.

2. Ferment at room temperature for 3 – 5 days. Store in the fridge for up to 3 months.

Yield: 16 Servings (2 T/serving)

Nutritional Information:

- Calories/serving: 11
- Net carbs: 1g
- Total Carbs: 2g
- Total Fat: 0g
- Fiber: 1g
- Protein: 0g

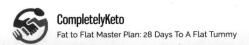

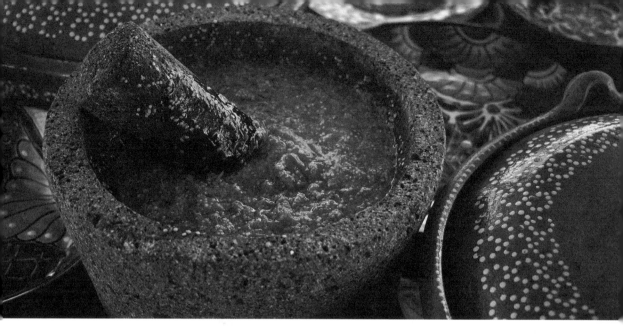

Fermented Red Salsa

Ingredients

- 4 medium tomatoes, small dice
- 1 yellow cooking onion, cut into large chunks
- 4 garlic cloves
- 1 small hot pepper, stem removed and cut in half
- 1 C cilantro
- Juice of 1 lime (about 2 T)
- 1 T pink Himalayan salt flakes

Preparation

1. Whiz tomatoes in blender or food processor and pour the crushed tomatoes into a bowl.

2. Place the remaining ingredients (except salt and lime juice) in the blender or food processor and pulse until finely chopped. Stir into the crushed tomato.

3. Add the lime juice and salt. Stir well and fill clean, wide mouth, pint-sized mason jar(s), tamping down the salsa so the liquid covers and submerges the salsa ingredients. Cover with a fermenting lid.

4. Allow the fermenting salsa to sit at room temperature for 3 – 5 days. Store in fridge for up to 3 months.

Yield: about 4 C (¼ C/serving)

Nutritional Information:

- Total Calories/serving: 11
- Total Carbs: 3g
- Fiber: 1g
- Net Carbs: 2g
- Total Fat: 0g
- Protein: 0g

CompletelyKeto
Fat to Flat Master Plan: 28 Days To A Flat Tummy

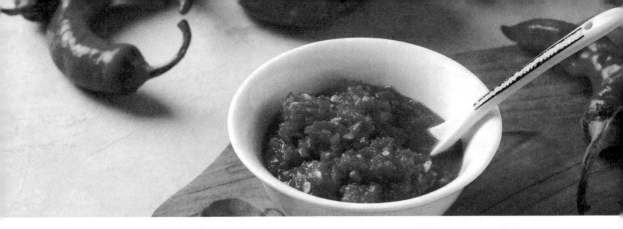

Fermented Hot Sauce

This gets prepped in minutes then Mother Nature finishes the work. Presto… fermented hot sauce is ready 5-7 days later! You can opt to replace some of the hot pepper with red bell pepper if you want a milder version. Don't worry if the hot sauce seems well … too hot, when first fermented. You will find it mellows after a few weeks in the fridge.

Ingredients

- 6 -7 C hot red chili peppers, stems removed and cut in half or into large chunks
- 4 garlic cloves, peeled
- 6 ¼ tsp fine sea salt
- 5 C filtered water

Preparation

1. Divide pepper chunks between two clean wide mouthed mason jars.
2. Make brine by adding salt to the water and swirling it around until the salt dissolves.
3. Pour brine into the jars so the peppers are just covered.
4. Use a ferment weight to keep the peppers submerged beneath the brine. Seal the jars, using a fermenting lid. Store in a cupboard for 7 days. If it's hot where you are then find a cooler spot in the basement out of the sun. Do a taste test at 5 days to see how they are doing. If you like the taste then the fermentation process is done.
5. Strain the peppers but save the brine. Place fermented peppers into the blender and process until you get the texture or smoothness you prefer. You can add some of the reserved brine as you blend if needed. Add some herbs or spices at this point again, if desired. Oregano, cumin and or ginger make nice additions.
6. Store in the fridge covered loosely with a lid that isn't screwed down tightly so gases can escape as the fermentation process will continue very slowly.

Yield: 8 Servings (about ¼ C/serving)

Nutritional Information:

- Calories/serving: 47
- Total Carbs: 10g
- Fiber: 2g
- Net carbs: 8g
- Total Fat: 1g
- Protein: 2g

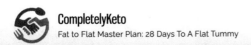

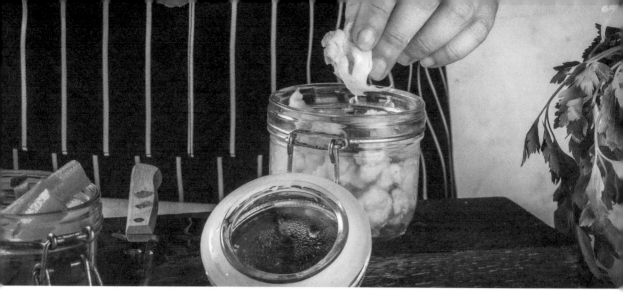

Fermented Cauliflower Pickles

These fermented pickles will be ready in 3-5 days and only take about 20 minutes to prep; easy to make and oh so tasty.

Ingredients

- 3 garlic cloves, peeled
- 4 C filtered water
- 2 T sea salt
- 1 head of cauliflower, cut into bite-sized florets and pieces

Preparation

1. Wash 3 wide mouth, pint sized glass Mason jars and place a peeled garlic clove in the bottom of each jar

2. Mix water and salt together and set aside.

3. Divide cauliflower between the jars and pour the brine over-top until the cauliflower is covered.

4. Place a glass ferment weight on top of the cauliflower so it is completely submerged in the brine.

5. Seal the jar with a fermenting lid if you have one, If not screw the lid on loosely and place the jars on a pan to catch drips which sometimes happen as the veggie ferments.

6. Do a taste test after 3 days. If you like the taste, the cauliflower is fermented enough and can be deemed done; if not leave for another few days.

Yield: 3 pints (about 24 cauliflower floret pickles)

Nutritional Information:

- Calories/serving: 7
- Total Carbs: 1g
- Fiber: 1g
- Net carbs: 0g
- Total Fat: 0g
- Protein: 0g

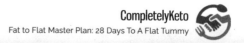

CompletelyKeto

Fat to Flat Master Plan: 28 Days To A Flat Tummy

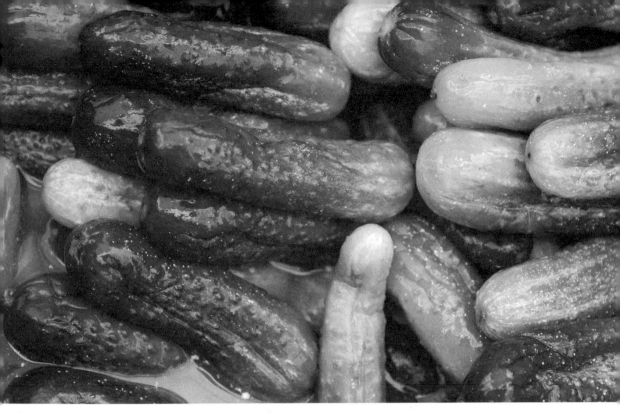

Fermented Sour Dill Pickles

These garlic/dill pickles taste like the old fashioned deli pickles that were available at the local butcher shop in my neighborhood, growing up.

Here are a few tips and things to watch for as your pickles ferment:

Kahm yeast, a thin white film, may develop on top of the pickles in the jar as they ferment. Don't worry it is normal and won't ruin this batch of pickles. Just carefully lift it off the top (it should stay intact) and discard the film.

The liquid in the jar will become cloudy and is simply a sign that fermentation is in progress.

The garlic cloves are full of anti-oxidants that tend to take on a bluish hue when fermented. No worries if your garlic is blue at the end of the fermenting process; this is normal!

Ingredients

- 4 C filtered water
- 2 T pink Himalayan salt flakes (or kosher salt flakes)
- 1 ½ lbs. pickling cucumbers
- 8 garlic cloves, peeled
- 1 tsp coriander seed
- 1 tsp mustard seed
- 1 dried chili pepper, optional
- 3 fresh, flowering dill heads, or ½ C of the finer dill leaves … or in a pinch use 3T dried dill

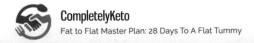

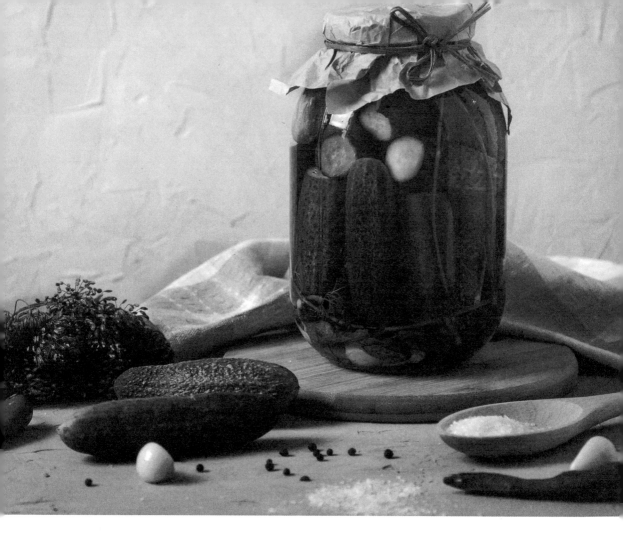

Preparation

1. Heat water in saucepan over high heat. Stir in the salt. Keep stirring until the salt dissolves then allow the liquid to cool down to room temperature before continuing.

2. While the brine is cooling, trim the stem end of cucumbers and cover them with cold water to refresh the cukes and crisp them up. This should take at least 20 minutes or maybe up to 1 hour. Drain and place into a clean jar. Add garlic, seeds and dill. Cover with the room temperature salt water and place a weight over-top. Seal with a fermenting lid. If using a regular lid "burp" the pickles daily to remove accumulated air and gases.

3. Ferment for at least one week. Does a taste test and if pickles are soured to your taste they are done. If not, continue the fermenting process for up to 2 months. Store in fridge when deemed done to your liking.

Yield: about 12 fermented pickles, 1 pickle per serving

Nutritional Information:

- Calories/serving: 4
- Net carbs: 1g
- Total Carbs: 1g
- Total Fat: 0g
- Fiber: 0g
- Protein: 0g

CompletelyKeto
Fat to Flat Master Plan: 28 Days To A Flat Tummy